Youth, AIDS and Sexually Transmitted Diseases

HIV/AIDS is a major life-threatening disease. It has caused a resurgence of concern about other sexually transmitted diseases (STDs) and their high rates among young people. This age group is increasingly sexually active, and at an increasingly early age.

Youth, AIDS and Sexually Transmitted Diseases reviews the current literature, research and educational and health policy concerning young people and STDs. It presents a comprehensive analysis of the impact of these diseases on young people, and examines how their sexual behaviour has changed as a result of the threat of AIDS. It looks at young people's knowledge and attitudes about their own sexual health, as well as the usefulness of models for predicting those at risk. Drawing on insights from their own research in the field, the authors also use the voices of young people to illustrate their concerns.

Youth, AIDS and Sexually Transmitted Diseases will be of considerable benefit to health care providers, sex educators, and all those who work with and study adolescents.

Susan Moore is Professor of Psychology at Victoria University of Technology, Melbourne, and co-author of *Sexuality in Adolescence* (1993) (with Doreen Rosenthal). Professor **Doreen Rosenthal** and **Anne Mitchell** are at the Centre for the Study of Sexually Transmissible Diseases, La Trobe University, Melbourne.

Adolescence and Society

Series editor: John C. Coleman
The Trust for the Study of Adolescence

The general aim of the series is to make accessible to a wide readership the growing evidence relating to adolescent development. Much of this material is published in relatively inaccessible professional journals, and the goals of the books in this series will be to summarise, review and place in context current work in the field so as to interest and engage both an undergraduate and a professional audience.

The intention of the authors is to raise the profile of adolescent studies among professionals and in institutions of higher education. By publishing relatively short, readable books on interesting topics to do with youth and society, the series will make people more aware of the relevance of the subject of adolescence to a wide range of social concerns.

The books will not put forward any one theoretical viewpoint. The authors will outline the most prominent theories in the field and will include a balanced and critical assessment of each of these. Whilst some of the books may have a clinical or applied slant, the majority will concentrate on normal development.

The readership will rest primarily in two major areas: the undergraduate market, particularly in the fields of psychology, sociology and education; and the professional training market, with particular emphasis on social work, clinical and educational psychology, counselling, youth work, nursing and teacher training.

Also available in this series

Identity in Adolescence
Jane Kroger

The Nature of Adolescence (second edition)
John C. Coleman and Leo Hendry

The Adolescent in the Family
Patricia Noller and Victor Callan

Young People's Understanding of Society
Adrian Furnham and Barrie Stacey

Growing up with Unemployment
Anthony H. Winefield, Marika Tiggermann, Helen R. Winefield and Robert D. Goldney

Young People's Leisure and Lifestyles
Leo B. Hendry, Janet Shucksmith, John G. Love and Anthony Glendinning

Sexuality in Adolescence
Susan Moore and Doreen Rosenthal

Adolescent Gambling
Mark Griffiths

Adolescent Health
Patrick C.L. Heaven

Youth, AIDS and Sexually Transmitted Diseases

Susan Moore, Doreen Rosenthal
and Anne Mitchell

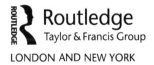

Routledge
Taylor & Francis Group

LONDON AND NEW YORK

Published 1996 by Routledge
27 Church Road, Hove, East Sussex BN3 2FA

Simultaneously published in the USA and Canada
by Routledge
711 Third Avenue New York, NY 10017

Routledge is an imprint of the Taylor & Francis Group, an informa business

© 1996 Susan Moore, Doreen Rosenthal, and Anne Mitchell

Typeset in Palatino by Routledge

Mackays of Chatham PLC, Chatham, Kent

British Library Cataloguing in Publication Data
A catalogue record for this book is available from the British
Library

Library of Congress Cataloguing in Publication Data
Moore, Susan, 1945–
Youth, AIDS, and sexually transmitted diseases / Susan
Moore, Doreen Rosenthal, and Anne Mitchell.
p. cm. — (Adolescence and society)
Includes bibliographical references and index.
1. AIDS (Disease) in adolescence — Social aspects. 2. Sexually
transmitted diseases — Social aspects. 3. Teenagers — Sexual
behavior. 4. Risk-taking (Psychology) in adolescence. 5. Safe
sex in AIDS prevention. I. Rosenthal, Doreen, 1938– . II.
Mitchell, Anne, 1946– . III. Title. IV. Series.
RJ387.A25M66 1996
616.95′1′00835 — dc20

96–11013
CIP

ISBN 13: 978-0-415-10633-7 (pbk)

To Ian, David, and Barbara

Contents

Notes on the authors   ix
Acknowledgements   xi
Introduction   xiii

1 **The scope of the problem: 'Taking a chance on love'**   1

2 **Youths' sexual behaviour**   16

3 **Understanding the risk: Young people's knowledge
   of and attitudes towards STDs**   35

4 **Predicting sexual risk taking: Theoretical frameworks**   53

5 **Myths and stereotypes: Young people's decisions to have
   and not to have safe sex**   72

6 **A matter of policy**   90

7 **Preventing STDs through education**   105

8 **Living with sexually transmissible disease**   126

9 **Conclusion**   144

References   149
Index   168

Notes on the authors

Susan Moore

Susan Moore holds the position of Inaugural Chair in Psychology at Victoria University of Technology. She holds a PhD from Florida State University, and BSc (Hons) and MEd degrees from the University of Melbourne. Her research is chiefly in the area of adolescent risk-taking and health, in particular adolescent sexual risk-taking and its implications with respect to HIV/AIDS. Professor Moore has held several major research grants, and published over fifty articles in refereed journals , as well as the book *Sexuality in Adolescence*, co-authored with Professor Doreen Rosenthal. She has worked as a school counsellor and taught in universities for over twenty-five years.

Doreen Rosenthal

Doreen Rosenthal is the Foundation Director of the Centre for the Study of Sexually Transmissible Diseases, La Trobe University, and Director of the Program in the General Community/Youth area of the National Centre in HIV Social Research. She holds a BA (Hons) and a PhD from the University of Melbourne. Professor Rosenthal is a developmental psychologist and an international expert in the field of adolescent sexuality. For the past seven years, Professor Rosenthal has been involved in a programme of research on adolescent risk-taking and HIV/AIDS. Her interests include gender and the social construction of sexuality. She is co-author, with Susan Moore, of *Sexuality in Adolescence*, and has published over a hundred articles on adolescent development.

Anne Mitchell

Anne Mitchell has a background in high-school teaching and adult education and has now been working in the field of HIV/AIDS education and sexual health for over ten years. She has worked in the policy development area of health promotion in the Victorian Health Department, and has a Master's degree in the area of women's health. Her current position is as Community Liaison Officer with the Centre for the Study of STDs at La Trobe University, where she has the responsibility of developing and maintaining effective links between researchers and the community. This involves the running of in-service education for teachers and health professionals, ensuring research outcomes are available in straightforward language for community members and organising public seminars and forums.

Acknowledgements

Many people have assisted in the process of bringing this book to fruition, not the least our colleagues, fellow researchers, and research assistants. We thank them all for their practical contributions, ideas, and encouragement. Special thanks are due to Heidi Reichler from the Centre for the Study of Sexually Transmissible Diseases, who collected together much of the research underpinning the *Young Heterosexuals, HIV/AIDS, and STDs* Report (Rosenthal and Reichler 1994), a document that formed the background for several of the chapters in this book. John Coleman, the editor of the series, also has our special thanks both for offering us the opportunity to write the book and for his patience in waiting for the manuscript.

We are appreciative that our employers, Victoria University of Technology and La Trobe University, provide an atmosphere of scholarship and practical facilities to enable a task such as this to be undertaken. Our own research is discussed frequently in the book, and it has provided a basis for our thinking about the issues associated with youth and sexually transmissible disease. The Commonwealth AIDS Research Grants Committee, Australia, and the Victorian Health Promotions Foundation have been consistent and generous in funding this research, and we are grateful for their support.

Most importantly, thanks go to the young people who have talked to us and whose experiences enrich the text and provide a framework for this book.

Introduction

HIV/AIDS is a new major life-threatening disease. It has caused a resurgence of concern about traditional sexually transmitted diseases and their high rates among young people, a concern that had, to some extent, been swept under the carpet in the pre-AIDS era. AIDS has forced us to consider new ways of thinking about sex, given the dangers inherent in practices that had become commonplace with the advent of the contraceptive pill and the higher levels of acceptance of both non-marital and non-heterosexual sex. However, recognition of the basic futility of attempting to ban socially tolerated behaviours, or turn back the clock, as a method of disease control has led to public health efforts to work with and modify these behaviours so that they can occur safely.

Young people have been one important target of these public-health interventions because of their particular vulnerabilities. As our book will show, this age group is increasingly sexually active, and at an increasingly early age. Many young boys and some girls report having multiple partners, and where they are in steady relationships these are by no means always sexually exclusive. If young people are faithful to one partner, this may be relatively (across a lifetime) short term with 'serial monogamy' – a succession of relationships, often of short-term duration – a common practice. As we shall further show, most sexually active young people are inconsistent or non-users of condoms, with some marginalised groups, such as the homeless and intravenous drug users, being particularly at risk because of their tendency towards high rates of unprotected intercourse, multiple partnering, and other risk behaviours.

In this book we review current literature, research, and policy concerning young people and sexually transmitted disease, with a particular emphasis on HIV/AIDS. Most of the research discussed derives from Western nations, simply because it is from these countries, particularly Britain, the United States, Canada, and Australia, that most publications emanate. Our findings and conclusions must therefore be viewed within this context. Understanding the spread of these diseases among young people in other cultural contexts, such as Asia or Africa, undoubtedly would require different sets of explanatory principles and models. The cultural embeddedness of our book is not denied. We argue though that the exercise of summarising and evaluating research and policy on youth and STDs within our own cultural context is a worthwhile one, as it provides, in a sense, a baseline for new research and new understandings to emerge. From such a position we can more readily decide where to go from here.

The aim of the book is to present a comprehensive and up-to-date analysis of the impact of STDs and, in particular, HIV on young people, within the cultural context described above. We hope that the book will be of use to policy makers, health care providers, sex educators, and others who work with and study adolescents and young people. Drawing insights from our own extended programmatic research in the field, we also use the voices of young people to illustrate their concerns and illuminate our understanding of their sexual world.

Chapter 1 contains a description and symptoms of various STDs, including HIV. Modes of transmission of these diseases are discussed, along with their incidence among young people, including regional variations in prevalence. Young people's sexual behaviour is described in Chapter 2, with sections on age of initiation, sexual experimentation and diversity, beliefs about faithfulness and monogamy, and incidence of unsafe sexual practices. Lifestyle factors of high-risk groups and their contribution to disease transmission are highlighted.

The basic questions discussed in Chapter 3 are 'What do young people know and think about STDs and precautions against them?' and 'Do young people perceive themselves to be at risk of STDs?' Research concerning young people's sources of information about these diseases and attitudes towards disease protection are presented.

In Chapter 4, models of behaviour used to explain risk taking, in particular sexual risk taking, among adolescents and youth are discussed. Examples of such models are the Theory of Reasoned Action and the Health Belief Model. The contributions and limitations of these models are reviewed. Chapter 5 comprises, for the most part, descriptions and evaluations of qualitative research concerning factors mitigating safe-sex practice. In this chapter we argue that theories of rational decision making can only go so far in predicting condom use and other safe-sex options among the young. It is vital that we also understand the social context of sexual behaviour and sexual relationships in order to predict (and ultimately influence) the uptake of safe-sex behaviours.

The issue of institutional policies concerning STDs and their relevance to the needs and behaviour of young people is addressed in Chapter 6. Confidentiality, service accessibility, and lack of discriminatory practices are considered as elements of good policy. The Australian experience as a model of effective action is reviewed. Chapter 7 concentrates on the role of education in preventing and managing STDs, with emphasis on the particular contributions of parents, the mass media and schools as agents of change. Current trends in peer education as an effective way of educating young people about safe and unsafe sexual practices are analysed in detail. In Chapter 8, the problems, issues and coping strategies of young people living with an STD, particularly HIV, are discussed.

Finally, in our concluding chapter, we address the question of whether the sexual behaviour and lifestyles of young people have changed as a result of the AIDS epidemic. We conclude that real and positive changes are occurring but at a slow rate, and that for some marginalised young people the dangers of sexually transmitted disease, and the curtailment of life's possibilities that these entail, are unacceptably high.

1 The scope of the problem
'Taking a chance on love'

It is unlikely that the writer of this popular song of the 1940s had syphilis or gonorrhoea in mind when he wrote it. Taking a chance on love then had a more innocent, less disturbing meaning than it does today. For today's young people, taking a chance on love has a potentially deadly or at least debilitating meaning. In this chapter we set the scene for the remainder of this book by describing some of the diseases that are sexually transmitted and the reasons why these diseases pose a special risk for adolescents.

A SHORT HISTORY

A short excursion into history reveals that concerns about sexual health and sexually transmissible diseases (STDs) are not new. Venereal diseases (VDs), to use an older term, have long been with us, waxing and waning as a public health issue over the centuries. For example, Waugh (1990) documents evidence of STDs from ancient Egyptian times to the modern day, with the establishment of the medical speciality of venereology. Some biblical descriptions of 'plague', where practices for preventing the contamination of others are specified, have been interpreted as references to venereal disease. The outbreak of syphilis in Europe in the fifteenth century began the thorough documentation of the history of this STD, and had a significant influence on public health measures as well as placing STDs within a moral context. Notification of syphilis became compulsory, and early in the sixteenth century it was decreed that syphilitics should lose their jobs. The moral condemnation surrounding syphilis continued into the nineteenth century, with syphilis being described in the 1867 edition of *Chambers Encyclopaedia* as 'this repulsive form of disease...usually propagated by impure sexual intercourse'. To this day, it is not unusual to hear syphilis and other

STDs being described as 'shameful' or 'dirty' even by young people (Smith *et al.* 1995).

The significance of syphilis and other STDs was often linked with its effects on soldiers and the war effort. In the same edition of *Chambers Encyclopaedia*, one Dr Aitken is quoted as observing that 'The loss of strength from venereal diseases … is equal to the loss of more than eight days annually of every soldier in service.' Another medical practitioner of the time, Dr Parkes, discusses the question of the prevention of syphilis. The means of prevention that he suggests are:

> (1) *Continence*, which is promoted by (a) the cultivation of a religious feeling and of pure thought and conversation; (b) the removal from temptation and occasions to sin; (c) constant and agreeable employment, bodily and mentally; and (d) temperance. (2) *Early marriage*. At present only six per cent of our soldiers are allowed to marry. (3) *Precautions after the risk of contagion*. In some French towns, the use of lotions and washing is rigorously enforced, with the effect of lessening the disease considerably. (4) *Cure of the disease in those affected by it*. Health inspections, in special reference to venereal disease, are made weekly in our army.
>
> (1867 edition of *Chambers Encyclopaedia*)

The First World War gave a great impetus to STD prevention, with all nations involved in the fighting taking measures to protect their troops. Taking Victoria, Australia, as a case study, notification of venereal disease was made compulsory at the time of the First World War and there was considerable, although often uninformed, concern about the widespread prevalence of these diseases. Of all the men examined during call-up in 1916, twenty in every 1,000 were found to be infected with gonorrhoea or syphilis. Other contemporary data show much higher estimates. There was an interesting slant to notions of prevention. The cause of VD was unequivocally attributed to women – prostitutes or 'scarlet women' of both the amateur and professional variety. The emphasis on dealing with syphilis at its cause, namely women, featured in Dr Parkes' writings in the mid-nineteenth century: 'Inspections of all recognised prostitutes have long been supported by legal authority.' Dr Parkes goes on to tell us that the Contagious Diseases Bill of 1864 allowed for diseased prostitutes found 'in the neighbourhood of certain places' to be taken into a hospital and detained there until cured. No such constraints appeared to apply to these women's infected partners. By whatever means, and for whatever reasons, by the Second World War the numbers infected with gonorrhoea or syphilis had dropped, although women were still targeted as the major cause of the evil.

By the 1990s, gonorrhoea and syphilis were no longer the most common, or even the most devastating, STDs. More prevalent today are chlamydia, genital warts and herpes, and, of course, the human immunodeficiency virus (HIV) and its outcome, acquired immune deficiency syndrome (AIDS). Since its detection in the West early in the 1980s, HIV/AIDS has quite properly become and remained a priority public-health issue. Nevertheless, the incidence of other STDs and their possible consequences makes it imperative that we cast our prevention strategies wider than the present focus on HIV and AIDS. In addition, it now seems that infection with HIV makes infection with another STD more likely, and the converse is also true.

The potential of AIDS to cut a swath through productive sectors of the population, especially the young, has served the important purpose of focusing attention on the sexual health of individuals in our society and placing this STD on the public health agenda. But it has also directed attention away from other STDs and their consequences to the health and well-being of the community. In the remainder of this chapter, we document some distinguishing features of a range of common modern STDs, including HIV/AIDS, and consider the risks these STDs carry for young people.

DESCRIBING STDs: WHAT ARE THE SYMPTOMS?

Any attempt to be comprehensive in describing STDs and their symptoms would leave the non-medical reader bewildered and overwhelmed. Instead, we focus on those STDs that appear to have most relevance to young people in the Western world, with the aim of briefly describing the symptoms they produce, and their possible complications. The interested reader is referred to detailed accounts in Adimara *et al.* (1994), Holmes *et al.* (1990), and Wasserheit *et al.* (1991). For a user-friendly discussion of signs, symptoms and consequences, the primer by Plummer *et al.* (1995) is recommended.

The microbiological agents responsible for most STDs are bacteria and viruses. Bacterial STDs such as gonorrhoea, chlamydia and syphilis can be cured, unlike viral STDs, such as HIV, genital herpes, or human papillomavirus (HPV). Individuals who become infected with these viruses usually remain so. For viral and some bacterial STDs there may be no overt manifestations of the disease so that the individual may be unaware that he or she is infected. The only STD for which an effective vaccine is available at present is hepatitis B virus.

Gonorrhoea

Commonly known as the 'clap', gonorrhoea (*Neisseria gonorrhoea*) is usually associated with a vaginal discharge in women and urethral discharge in men, but there can be infection in the throat, the upper genital tract in women (uterus or fallopian tubes) or in the rectum, and pain on urinating is common. There has been a significant decrease in the number of cases of gonorrhoea in many Western countries, partly as a consequence of greater awareness of safe-sex issues. Mindel (1995) reports that in those countries where there has been a decrease in gonorrhoea, there has also been a significant increase in pelvic inflammatory disease and ectopic pregnancies. About 50 per cent of all women and between 1 and 3 per cent of men infected are asymptomatic and reinfections are common.

The organism cannot survive for a long period outside the human host and is most commonly spread through sexual intercourse. Jones and Wasserheit (1991) report that the chance of a woman who has intercourse with an infected man being infected is between 50 and 90 per cent, depending on the number of exposures. A single exposure from an infected woman results in a 20 per cent chance of a man becoming infected, with that chance increasing with subsequent exposure.

Treatment is safe and highly effective, the preferred option being single-dose regimes. Such quick, short-term treatment is more likely to be followed by patients than long-term alternatives.

Chlamydia trachomatis infections

Chlamydia infections are of particular concern because of their prevalence and the high likelihood that infection will be asymptomatic. Infections usually involve the same sites as those infected by gonorrhoea but are less acute and produce milder symptoms, or no discernible symptoms. Infections of the eye may result from contact with genital secretions. Estimates are that of those infected, 90 per cent of women and 50 to 90 per cent of men are asymptomatic. Because of this, early treatment (or indeed any treatment) is often not sought and, as a consequence, complications of chlamydia are common.

Transmission from one person to another is through sexual intercourse, and recurrent infections are common. About two-thirds of women and one-third of men with infected partners become infected themselves (Jones and Wasserheit 1991).

Diagnosis is best made through tissue culture although other less sensitive tests are available. Treatment is usually effective, although the need for multiple dose therapy means that compliance is often difficult to achieve and another major barrier to treatment is the difficulty of diagnosis.

Genital herpes

Genital herpes is a chronic disease, of which there are two types: herpes simplex virus type 1 (HSV1), which is commonly associated with the cold sore blister, and type 2 (HSV2), which occurs around the genital region and is usually associated with genital herpes. However, both HSV1 and HSV2 can infect either site. It has been suggested that genital infection caused by HSV1 infections are increasing as a result of an increasing awareness of safer sex practices with respect to HIV infection, and thus an increase in oral–genital sex.

Symptoms are, initially, a period of discomfort characterised by hypersensitivity. Within one to three days, lesions develop to form painful superficial ulcers. Other symptoms may include fever, headache and a feeling of tiredness. The symptoms of primary infection persist for one to three weeks. The lymph nodes may be enlarged and tender for up to six weeks. Clinical manifestations of the infection will depend on the site of entry and any immunity acquired from a previous attack. Recurrent infections are less severe and shorter. Jones and Wasserheit (1991) report that individuals infected with HSV2 are almost twice as likely to have one or more recurrent infections within 12 months of first being infected than those infected with HSV1 (about 90 per cent of cases compared with 50 per cent). Corey (1990) reports a two-year follow-up study in which the median recurrence rate was five episodes per year. While there are periods of latency, relapses tend to occur when the individual is subjected to emotional or physical stress, fever, hormonal changes, or a number of other factors.

Diagnosis is relatively easy when the individual is symptomatic. In the absence of symptoms, viral cultures are necessary. There is no cure for genital herpes although antiviral therapy can shorten the duration of the primary infection and suppress recurrent infection. However, as Jones and Wasserheit note, when therapy ceases, recurrences of the infection occur at the same rate as previously.

A major problem with genital herpes is that the virus may be shed in the absence of obvious symptoms so that a person can be infected or infectious without realising it. In fact, Mindel (1995) argues that close questioning of most infected individuals reveals that they do have genital symptoms which neither they nor their doctors recognise as being due to genital herpes. Indeed, Mindel estimates that 60 per cent of infected people have unrecognised symptoms and only 20 per cent are asymptomatic. Fortunately, at least one study has shown that transmission rates are relatively low (Mertz *et al.* 1988).

Genital warts

Genital warts (resulting from infection with human papillomavirus) are contracted, as a rule, through direct sexual contact, and it is not uncommon for other STDs to be present concurrently (Oriel 1990). Infections with HPV are common (Mindel 1995) and the incidence of genital warts appears to have increased despite the use of safe-sex techniques. The reasons for this may be the lengthy incubation period for HPV infection, the asymptomatic nature of many infections, and that using condoms (the most preferred and most promoted safe-sex technique) does not cover all the areas that are likely to be exposed to the wart virus. Most people with genital warts have no symptoms and concern usually is with appearance of the warts. The virus manifests itself about two months after infection (or any time between one and six months). Initially there may be reddish swellings that grow into a cluster of small, painless, cauliflower-shaped lumps on the penis, perineum, labia, vulva, cervix, or in and around the anus. In men, warts may be infrequently located on the scrotum or urethra. Cervical lesions tend not to be warty. If occurring in the vagina or anus, warts may go undetected. Infection may also occur without the development of actual warts.

The likelihood of being infected after a single exposure is not known, but two studies reported by Oriel suggest moderately high levels of infectivity, with about two-thirds of the sex partners of infected individuals with genital warts developing the disease. There are various treatments for genital warts, such as electrocautery (heat) under local anaesthetic, the application of liquid nitrogen (cold), or antiviral therapy. Estimates are that only about 25 per cent of people with warts are cured and although it has been suggested that warts will disappear spontaneously, there is little evidence for this claim.

Hepatitis B (HBV)

Hepatitis B affects the functioning of the liver, and infection with HBV may, uncommonly, lead to death from acute or chronic liver failure or liver cancer. Sexual activity is a major factor in the transmission of HBV, especially for homosexual men, although other routes of infection are common. Lemon and Newbold (1990) suggest that many adults infected with HBV have silent infections which probably result in permanent immunity. The onset of HBV is generally insidious, with an incubation period of about six weeks before onset of symptoms. The initial symptoms include fever, rash, and painful joints. There may be some jaundice causing yellowing of the skin and whites of the eyes. As HBV is a disease affecting the liver, there may be dark urine. Jones and Wasserheit report that only about one-third of infected adults are diagnosed clinically as having viral hepatitis, one-third have mild symptoms, and one-third are asymptomatic. Most patients recover completely, usually within six to eight weeks, although some individuals may develop chronic Hepatitis B, become a permanent carrier (more likely in the young), or develop cirrhosis.

Sexual transmission of HBV is strongly linked with number of partners and the practice of anal intercourse. Moderate rates of transmission are reported from an infected to an uninfected partner (about 18 to 27 per cent in heterosexual couples, with substantially higher rates for homosexual men).

Although there is no effective cure for HBV, there is a vaccine that provides immunity for most individuals for a period up to two years, although for some people protection for five years is possible.

Human immunodeficiency virus (HIV)

Although HIV is believed to have been spreading in Africa from the 1940s, it was not officially recognised until 1981, when the Center for Disease Control in the USA set up a task force to investigate reports of an unusual immune deficiency disease in a growing number of gay men. Its early title of gay-related immune deficiency (GRID) reflects this history, and it was retitled AIDS (acquired immune deficiency syndrome) in 1982 when increasing numbers of non-gay infected people emerged, mainly intravenous drug users. The 1984 discovery, by both French and American scientists, of the human immunodeficiency virus that causes AIDS was the beginning of a real understanding of how the disease was transmitted and how it would need to be prevented.

This is not the place to present a full picture of the biology, clinical manifestations, and treatment of HIV (see Holmes *et al.* 1990 for a full description). The virus attacks the cells of the immune system, eventually causing AIDS, and can be transmitted in one of three ways: through sexual contact with an infected person, by a pregnant woman to the foetus or after birth during breast feeding, and through exposure to contaminated blood (sharing needles and syringes that are contaminated, through needle-stick injuries, or through blood transfusions). Many individuals have no or very mild symptoms at the time of infection. However, in some, there is an influenza-like episode, and neurological signs may be present, including severe headaches, stiff neck, or more serious symptoms. The illness lasts about two to three weeks but there is usually full recovery. An infected person may remain asymptomatic for a variable period, with absence of symptoms now reported for periods of up to twelve years among some individuals. Plummer and his colleagues report that about one-third to half of those who have been infected with HIV for nine years will have developed AIDS (Plummer *et al.* 1995).

Early symptoms of AIDS are varied and include chronic fever, night sweats, diarrhoea, oral thrush, weight loss and herpes. The term ARC (AIDS-related complex) is sometimes used to characterise an early stage of AIDS with the presence of several symptoms. The development of AIDS is heralded by a range of conditions, including opportunistic infections, malignancies (such as Karposi's sarcoma), wasting syndrome, and severe neurological symptoms.

The virus is detected through HIV antibody testing. There is a 'window' period of about three months when the test will produce a negative result despite presence of the virus. Because the virus cannot be destroyed, infection lasts for life and can be passed on to others. We now know that the periods of greatest infectivity are at the time of becoming first infected or seroconversion (when tests may prove to be falsely negative) and at the time of transition to AIDS. While, at present, the onset of AIDS is an inevitable consequence of HIV infection, there are a number of strategies to improve or maintain general health. These include attending to diet, physical fitness, reduction of stress, and treatment of infections. Several therapeutic strategies are currently being tested, although at present there is no vaccine available and no cure for HIV/AIDS. Treatment with antiviral drugs such as Zidovudine may delay the onset of AIDS, decrease mortality, and reduce the number of opportunistic infections. At present, it appears that a combination of drugs may yield the best therapeutic results. Nevertheless, available data suggest that we are still far from finding a medical way to prevent HIV infection and that we need to focus on behaviour change so that transmission can be avoided.

The high morbidity and mortality associated with HIV, the fact that there is no cure and that, once infected, an individual is infected for life, places HIV/AIDS in a specially disturbing category among STDs. There also appears to be a link between HIV and other STDs. There is growing evidence (see Adimara *et al.* 1994) that other STDs, especially gonorrhoea, increase the risk of HIV infection (three- to five-fold by one estimate, Wasserheit 1992). Moreover, HIV infection appears to increase the prevalence of some STDs. As Short (1993) notes: 'Since these STDs in turn also increase the incidence of HIV infection, we have a true "epidemiological synergy", with each infection exacerbating the other' (Short 1993: 2). This relationship is one that can only highlight the need to address *all* STDs if we are to be effective in reducing the impact of HIV infection.

WHAT ARE THE COMPLICATIONS OF STD?

For most STDs, not only HIV, there is the possibility of distressing and debilitating, even fatal, complications. We have discussed above the fatal complications of chronic HBV, namely cirrhosis of the liver or cancer of the liver. In the remainder of this section we focus on other disturbing outcomes of STDs, not all of which are necessarily fatal.

One of the more common sequelae of gonorrhoea or chlamydia is pelvic inflammatory disease (PID). While STDs are not the only cause of PID, they are a major factor in many cases. In turn, PID is a significant cause of fertility problems in men and women. Plummer *et al.* (1995) cite Swedish research that shows that 11 per cent of women who have a single attack of PID are likely to become infertile. After two attacks, 23 per cent will be infertile, and after three attacks, 54 per cent of women will be unable to conceive. So, what is PID and how do you know that you have it?

In women, PID involves infection of the uterus, the Fallopian tubes and the lining of the pelvic organs. PID often has no symptoms, although sometimes there will be a vaginal discharge or burning when passing urine early on. Later symptoms may include pain in the abdomen, pain when having sex, changes in menstrual patterns and, possibly, fever. Untreated, PID can result in infertility, ectopic pregnancy and chronic pelvic pain. Yet, if diagnosed, PID can be treated easily and effectively with antibiotics – the difficulty often is in making the diagnosis in the absence of symptoms.

Further possible consequences of STD infections are also serious. There is evidence that precancerous abnormalities in the cervix are associated with sexual activity, probably through the introduction of infection. In particular, it is commonly accepted that genital warts are related to subsequent development of cancer of the cervix. While it is important that every woman has regular screening for cell abnormalities, it is particularly important that once warts are detected, women have regular Pap smears, preferably every six months.

In addition to the direct effects of STDs on women, there is the possibility of mother-to-child infection and other complications for the infant of an infected mother during pregnancy and birth. Infection can occur when bacteria or viruses pass from the mother's blood to the foetus's blood during pregnancy. Several STDs, including syphilis and HBV, can be transmitted in this way, as can HIV. At the present time, about one-quarter of babies born to women who are HIV-positive are found to be infected with HIV after birth. Unfortunately, there is no known treatment, in the cases of HIV or HBV, that will prevent infection of the baby during pregnancy. It is now known that breast feeding is a transmission route for HIV from mother to infant.

STD organisms can also be transmitted to the baby as it passes through an infected birth canal. In particular, gonorrhoea can cause eye infections that may result in blindness in the infant. Chlamydia is another STD that can be transmitted in this way. About 70 per cent of infants born to women with chlamydia acquire the infection at the time of birth. Eye infections are a common complication but, unlike the conjunctivitis caused by gonorrhoea, chlamydial conjunctivitis, which occurs in 20 to 30 per cent of neonates, has no long-term consequences.

Transmission of the virus causing genital warts may occur from mother to infant during birth, although with relatively low frequency. Of considerably more concern are the consequences of maternal–infant transmission of herpes, although estimates of transmission by this mode are low. (Jones and Wasserheit (1991) report that the incidence of neonatal infections is 1 in 2,000 to 1 in 5,000 deliveries per year in the United States.) Infants may be infected at or before birth and these infections are often fatal or lead to complications such as severe brain damage. Primary infection can cause spontaneous abortion, foetal abnormality, or prematurity. Recurrent infection is usually associated with infection at the time of birth.

Most textbooks on STDs emphasise these serious complications, both to the primary infected person and, in the case of women of child-bearing age, possible consequences for the foetus. Plummer *et al.* (1995) usefully draw our attention to a different set of outcomes, which they class as sexual dysfunction. We would wish to add to this outcome that of 'relationship dysfunction'. Diagnosis of an STD is, for most people, a disturbing and distressing event and one that requires certain changes in their lives. These changes not only involve the person who has the STD but also have important implications for his or her sexual partner or partners and present or future relationships. Being diagnosed with an STD may cause considerable problems for the continuation of a relationship because the person who is infected may be concerned about infecting his or her partner, or fear rejection by a current or potential partner.

The psychological problems associated with diagnosis of an STD, especially one for which there is no known cure, have been little studied and yet have the potential to hinder severely the ability of the individual to live a normal life. At the very least, sexual activity has to be monitored and negotiated while the person is infected. Even following treatment and, possibly but not always, cure, some individuals may find it difficult to resume their normal sexual lives. Impotence, or loss of interest in and enjoyment of sex, is an outcome that may require the services of a counsellor to overcome. Of course, for those STDs for which there is no cure, there are major life-long adjustments to be made, both for the individual infected and for his or her sexual partner or partners. Anger at being infected, anxiety about resuming sexual relationships, depression, even suicidal thoughts are not uncommon outcomes. All of these need to be recognised and dealt with, a process that can be assisted by trained counsellors.

DIFFICULT OR EASY TO CATCH?

The frequency and distribution of STDs (the *epidemiology* of these diseases) reflect people's patterns of sexual behaviour and the networks of sexual partners that they have. In general, STD rates are higher in men than women, among urban dwellers, and youth. However, as many writers note (see, for example, Aral and Holmes 1990), it is difficult to obtain accurate data about the frequency and distribution of STDs. Not all STDs are reportable, diagnosis may not be accurate, and many are asymptomatic as we have noted. There are also shifts in the incidence of STDs over time and across populations. For example, Aral and Holmes (1990) note that there was a steady increase in the incidence of viral STDs and chlamydial infections in Europe and North America during the 1970s and 1980s, with declines in the incidence of gonorrhoea and syphilis (but note the resurgence of these STDs in parts of the United States in the late 1980s and 1990s, associated with a crack cocaine epidemic). These shifts, however, were not uniform from country to country. Even within countries, there are sub-populations that may be more (or less) affected. In the United States, race and socioeconomic status are important indicators, together with age.

Whatever the changing patterns of STD incidence may be, it is clear that youth is a 'risk factor' for transmission. Stevenson *et al.* (1992) report that studies world-wide show that young people are at high risk for STDs. They report data from the United States that show that the highest rates of gonorrhoea and chlamydia occur among 15- to 19-year-olds. In that country, STDs disproportionately affect the health of adolescents. A recent report (Ellickson *et al.* 1993) included STDs among the major causes of mortality and morbidity for adolescents, claiming that approximately 86 per cent of all STDs occur among young people between the ages of 15 and 29 years. Infection rates for chlamydia were as high as 37 per cent of adolescents among some populations studied and national data showed that, in 1989, young people between the ages of 10 and 19 accounted for 30 per cent of new gonorrhoea cases, amounting to over 215,000 cases of gonorrhoea. The report concludes that, overall, approximately one in five adolescents will have acquired a sexually transmitted disease by the time he or she is 21 years old. Short (1993) reported that, in 1980, about one in every 100 women in the United States aged 15 to 19 who had ever had sex was hospitalised for pelvic inflammatory disease.

Surveillance data for 1992 in Victoria, Australia (Stevenson 1993), indicate that males in the 13- to 24-year age group represented 27 per cent and females almost 50 per cent of gonorrhoea cases, 31 per cent of male and 43 per cent of female acute hepatitis B infections, and 40 per cent of male and 67 per cent of female cases of non-specific urethritis or genital chlamydia infections. In the same report, rates of genital herpes and genital warts indicate that young people are vulnerable, with 13- to 24-year-olds providing 23 per cent of diagnoses of herpes and 39 per cent of diagnoses of genital warts. These high rates of chlamydial infection among adolescents are confirmed in other Australian states (Hart 1993). Finally, in a prospective study of the prevalence of chlamydia in young sexually active women, Kovacs and his colleagues found that women who gave positive results for chlamydia were younger than those who had negative results (Kovacs *et al.* 1987). Garland *et al.* (1993) confirm that young age is a risk factor for acquiring chlamydial infections.

Of concern is the evidence for an increase in the number of diagnosed cases of STDs among young people. For example, in 1966 in the United States, there were 50,000 reported cases of genital warts. By 1989 this figure had risen to 300,000 (Cates 1991). Similar worrying increases have been reported for genital herpes. It is not our intention here to undertake a full and thorough analysis of world-wide epidemiological data. Nevertheless, while we do not have available evidence for similar dramatic increases in other countries (and in Australia, where we have examined the transmission data, these are both too recent and too incomplete to be of great use to us here), there seems to be little doubt on the part of most epidemiologists that young people are significantly at risk of becoming infected with most STDs, relative to their older (and younger) peers.

The picture is somewhat different when we turn to HIV infection. The terrifying nature of the HIV/AIDS pandemic is apparent when we look at World Health Organization (WHO) estimates of the current numbers of infected people, and people with AIDS. The latter estimate is that there are 4.5 million people, world-wide, with AIDS. In total, 19.5 million people have been infected with HIV since the late 1970s and about 13 to 15 million of these are still alive. What is particularly worrying is the jump in new infections. We are not seeing an epidemic that is dying, or winding down.

According to the WHO, Africa accounts for about 70 per cent of the people infected with AIDS. In 1990 it was estimated that one in forty Africans was infected with HIV; two years later, that estimate was 20 per cent of 20- to 40-year-olds in many countries. What has happened in Africa is now happening in Asia, but at a faster pace. In the past year, infections have increased eight-fold in Asia. Again, the WHO estimates that the Asian region has about 3 million people who are infected with the AIDS virus.

Although it is estimated that over half the world's infections occur in 15- to 24-year-olds and most deaths from AIDS occur among those in the 20- to 40-year group, the patterns of infection world-wide differ substantially. While the transmission route is mainly by heterosexual contact in Africa and Asia, homosexual contact is the most common source of infection in many Western countries. In other countries, or cities, injecting drug users, whether heterosexual or homosexual, are the most likely sources of infection. Teenagers represent only a small proportion (under 1 per cent) of the total number of AIDS cases reported in the United States, Europe and Australia and, in Australia, only 2.1 per cent of those infected with HIV (Bury 1991; DiClemente 1992; National Centre in HIV Epidemiology and Clinical Research 1994). In spite of these apparently low figures, AIDS is the sixth leading cause of death for persons aged between 15 and 24 years in the United States, and the number of teenagers infected with HIV increased by 70 per cent in the two years between 1990 and 1992 (Haffner 1992).

We conclude this section by noting that age (specifically adolescence) is denoted as a risk marker or risk factor for STDs in most texts on the topic (see, for example, Aral and Holmes 1990; Wasserheit *et al.* 1991). The reasons for this are many and varied, ranging from the biological vulnerability of adolescents (Brookman 1990) to psychosocial factors and, specifically, the social environment in which young people develop and become mature sexual beings.

TAKING THE FIRST STEPS

One of the difficulties in treating STDs among young people is their frequent reluctance to present for treatment even when they suspect that they may be infected. There are many reasons for this, including anxiety about the diagnosis, concerns about confidentiality, lack of finance, and difficulties of access to health professionals. However, for those young people who do seek diagnosis and treatment, there are a number of key messages (Adimara *et al.* 1994).

First, compliance with the treatment regimen is essential. It is easy to forget to take medication, to avoid taking medication because of unwanted side effects, or to become confused about complex regimens. Second, for specific STDs, follow-up tests are critical. These follow-up tests are important for control of STDs and for ensuring that the treatment regime is maintained.

A young person who is infected has a responsibility not to infect knowingly his or her partner. This can be achieved by engaging in 'safe sex' (using condoms or non-penetrative sexual practices) or by deciding to abstain from sex while infected. It is essential that partners of infected individuals are identified and examined in order to reduce the likelihood of reinfection. Identification and referral for treatment of partners can occur in several ways. The infected person can notify all of his or her sexual partners of the possibility that they may be infected and should be examined. Or this can be done by contact tracing, where the patient provides information to health professionals about his or her sexual partners, who may then be contacted and requested to report for testing.

It is also important that young people respond quickly to any suspicion that they may be infected. Given that the symptoms of some STDs are mild or even absent, it may be difficult to know when one is infected. Lack of symptoms is not a guide to being disease free so that young people must be alert to the possibility of becoming infected by having unprotected sex with an infected partner. Unhappily, continued unprotected sexual activity while infected, whether knowingly or not, will contribute to the spread of STDs.

Having alerted people to the need for a quick and complete response to the suspicion of infection with an STD, it is perhaps timely to note that mistakes in diagnosis can be made, depending on the skill of the practitioner and the sophistication of the test used. Tests are not infallible, so a clinical examination is essential, and anxiety about symptoms may be unwarranted. Plummer and his colleagues make a point of reassuring worried readers that not all vaginal discharges or urinary problems denote the presence of an STD, but may be due to a mild loss of bladder control, in the former case, or bladder infections in the latter. What appear to be warts in the genital region may be normal structures such as fleshy tags on the penis, hair follicles, akin to 'goose bumps', or blocked sebaceous glands which may result in cysts.

Knowing that accurate diagnosis is sometimes difficult, that compliance with medication is not guaranteed, and that there are many individuals with 'silent' infections, protection from infection is dependent on persuading young people to avoid risky sexual practices. How this message is communicated and the factors that influence risk taking are an important focus of this book.

2 Youths' sexual behaviour

What do you think of sex before marriage?

I have been brought up as a good Catholic, that it is sinful and disgusting; but I have my own personal view that you have to. You don't just walk into a shop with your eyes shut and pick the clothing off the rack and take it home and open your eyes and see it is disgusting. You should sample before you buy. I guess it is just peer group pressure – you get to a stage where your hand gets boring. You want real flesh and meat and bone.

How is a casual sexual relationship different from romantic love?

A casual relationship, you are not really involved, you are just after sex and a bit of fun. Whereas romantic love is a more long-term, steady relationship – someone with a bit more care. There would be more communication with the romantic love partner. You'd find out each other's feelings and stuff.

Will AIDS affect how you go about sex in the future?

Yes, probably. You will have to be more careful. As you get older it will be more of a worry.

In some ways, these quotations from three 16-year-old boys sum up the 'modal' adolescent view of sex – premarital sex is the norm, casual and steady relationships have different rules, and worry about AIDS is something for the future. But of course that is oversimplifying and, as this chapter will show, there is a great deal of diversity among young people in their sexual behaviours and level of risk.

Obtaining information about the nature and extent of young people's sexual practices can be difficult, since schools (and parents) are often reluctant to have intimate and sensitive questions about sexuality asked of young adolescents. As a result, university or college students are regularly targeted for such studies. While there is, therefore, a considerable amount of information now available on late adolescents, there are few studies that target young teenagers. Ironically, given their higher rates of infection with STDs, there are even fewer studies that focus specifically on the post-teenage population in their early twenties.

There is also variation in the questions asked of young people with regard to their sexual practices. In earlier studies, and in some recent ones because of limitations placed on researchers by schools or institutions, details of specific practices (for example, oral, vaginal and anal sex) were not sought, nor were there attempts to differentiate practices with casual or regular sexual partners. The importance of obtaining detailed information about specific practices and partners is now recognised, but the different reporting practices make comparisons difficult. With these caveats in mind, we turn to the research findings.

SEXUAL DEBUT

A trend towards first experience of sex at younger ages is true of most Western countries (Goldman and Goldman 1988). In Sweden, the age of initiation into sex dropped from an average of 19 years to 16 years over the past four decades. British studies suggest similar data, with Breakwell and Fife-Schaw's (1992) survey of over 2,000 16- to 20-year-olds indicating that about 55 per cent of 16- to 17-year-olds had had vaginal intercourse at least once. The British *Sexual Attitudes and Lifestyles* survey of approximately 19,000 randomly selected individuals showed the median age of first intercourse of the youngest cohort sampled (16- to 24-year-olds), to be 17 years, some four years earlier than first intercourse of the oldest cohort (55 to 59 years) (Johnson *et al.* 1994). Hofferth *et al.* (1987) report that the majority of US teenagers have had sexual intercourse by the age of 19 years. They note, on the basis of their national survey, that by age 15, about 6 per cent of girls and 17 per cent of boys had experienced intercourse, these figures rising to 44 per cent and 67 per cent respectively by age 18, and to 70 and 80 per cent by age 20. Comparisons with Kinsey's early data lead us to conclude that while the average age of sexual debut has reduced somewhat for boys over the past forty years or so, the change is much more dramatic for girls, particularly Caucasian girls (Kinsey *et al.* 1948, 1953). American writers report these changes as gaining momentum in the mid-1970s, having arisen from the more sexually permissive attitudes of the 1960s and 1970s (Brooks-Gunn and Furstenberg 1989; Dusek 1991; Hofferth and Hayes 1987).

The Australian Institute of Family Studies conducted research in the early 1980s, which indicated that the move towards earlier sexual debut may have occurred later in Australia. At this time (1981–2), 60 per cent of 17-year-olds were still virgins, while in 1988, this had dropped to 40 per cent (Goldman and Goldman 1988). Research using a cross-national Australian sample of nearly 4,000 high school students was conducted by the National Centre in HIV Social Research in 1992 (Dunne *et al.* 1993a). In response to the question 'Have you ever had sex?', approximately half the boys and girls in year 12 (17- and 18-year-olds) responded in the affirmative. This number decreased steadily in lower age groups, although 13.5 per cent of boys and 6.5 per cent of girls in year 7 (12- and 13-year-olds) reported that they had had sex. The majority of students had had only one partner in the previous year; however, nearly one-third of year 12 boys and one-fifth of year 12 girls reported having had sex with three or more partners in that period.

It is somewhat misleading to talk of an average age for loss of virginity. There are considerable cultural and sub-group differences among young people. Studies from a range of countries indicate different levels of sexual experience for similarly aged young people from different social, religious, ethnic and racial groups. For example, black American adolescents become sexually active at a younger age than whites, and are more likely to be having sex than whites across the ages 11 to 17 (Bauman and Udry 1981; Newcomer and Udry 1983; Zelnick *et al.* 1981). Several studies note the lower rates of adolescent sexual intercourse (and the later ages of sexual debut), of Mexican-Americans in comparison with their Anglo-American counterparts (Aneshensel *et al.* 1989; Slonim-Nevo 1992). Adherence to religious values has generally been found to be negatively related to premarital sexual behaviour, with religious persons of all denominations less likely to be sexually active (Devaney and Hubley 1981; Spanier 1976). A significant number of young people advocate no sex before marriage, and although it is difficult to assess how many act on this, it appears that perhaps 15 to 20 per cent of 20-year-olds may have not yet experienced intercourse (e.g. Rogel *et al.* 1980; Rosenthal *et al.* 1990). A recent movement in the United States, the True Love Waits campaign, is apparently gaining popularity with particular sections of the teenage community. Their 'pledge' is:

Believing that true love waits, I make a commitment to God,

myself, my family, my friends, my future mate, and my future children to be sexually abstinent from this day until I enter a biblical marriage relationship.

(Henry 1995: 42)

At the other extreme, prepubertal intercourse occurs among a small but significant proportion of young people, often as a result of sexual abuse (Weber *et al.* 1989). The Goldmans (1988), for example, found that 8 per cent of children reported the transition from virgin to non-virgin between 10 and 13 years of age. Recent research with about 300 18-year-old intravenous drug users (IDUs) (Louie *et al.* 1996) found that sexual intercourse began at an earlier age for this group than reported for their non-IDU peers. The mean age of first intercourse in this IDU group was around 14 years, an age at which most studies of young people report only low levels of sexual activity.

Our interviews with young people suggest that the majority of adolescents themselves believe that 15 is too young an age to begin intercourse, and although the ideal age for loss of virginity 'depends on the person' (their level of maturity), too early sexual debut can have a damaging psychological effect. Nevertheless the belief that first sex should wait for marriage is no longer widely held (Moore and Rosenthal 1992b). Perhaps the most common view of young people today can be summed up in the words of a 16-year-old girl interviewed in an Australian study of adolescent sexual attitudes (Buzwell *et al.* 1992).

It's normal to have sex before marriage. No one waits for the ring these days. That idea is so old-fashioned. No one thinks like that anymore.

A popular modification of this attitude, presented by a different girl from the same study, mirrors research findings from Britain and the USA indicating that young people on the whole prefer to be sexually active within a committed relationship (e.g. Coleman and Hendry 1990; Dusek 1991). At face value these idealistic attitudes would appear to support safe-sex practices, but, paradoxically, in some situations they do not, an issue that is discussed further in Chapter 5.

I think I am a pretty modern girl. I don't believe that you actually have to be married. But you can't just do it with anyone. It has to be someone you really love and trust. Someone you have been seeing for a really long time.

SEXUAL EXPERIMENTATION AND DIVERSITY

Variety of practices

Current data, both qualitative (Stancombe 1994) and quantitative, suggest that young people are engaging in a wide variety of sexual behaviours. The variety reflects a generational change. Johnson *et al.* (1994) note that while the experience of vaginal intercourse is almost universal in Britain by age 25, there are marked age differences in other practices, particularly cunnilingus and fellatio. In the youngest age group studied (16–24 years), among those who had ever had vaginal sex, 79 per cent reported oral sex in the last year and 85 per cent ever, in comparison with, for example the 45 to 49 cohort for whom only 30 per cent of the women and 42 per cent of the men had had oral sex in the last year. These lower rates were sustained in the 'ever' category as well, with only half the women and two-thirds of the men over 45 having experienced oral sex in their lifetime. Johnson *et al.* (1994) note that these age differences in practice are reflected in other studies as well, and that there is a significant proportion of young people now for whom the practice of oral sex precedes coitus (Coles and Stokes 1985). Newcomer and Udry (1985), in a survey of adolescents in the USA, found that 25 per cent of virgin boys and 15 per cent of virgin girls had given or received oral–genital stimulation.

These findings are reflected in Australian studies. Roberts *et al.* (1996) report that the majority of their first-year university students had engaged in oral sex at least once, while 78 per cent of sexually active students had both given and received oral sex. Oral sex was common with regular partners among the tertiary students in Rosenthal *et al.*'s study (1990), with only 23 per cent of the sample never having engaged in this practice.

Thus the practice of oral sex appears widespread among adolescents, occurring frequently with regular partners and somewhat less so with casual partners. Interestingly, while oral sexual practices are potentially less risky than vaginal intercourse with respect to AIDS transmission, oral intercourse has been implicated in HIV transmission (Spitzer and Weiner 1989), and a range of STDs can be spread by these practices, particularly if semen, blood or vaginal fluids enter the mouth (Victorian Government Department of Health and Community Services 1993).

The incidence of anal sex, while relatively low, occurs with more frequency among some groups and more often with regular than with casual partners. About 3 per cent of a sample of heterosexual university students tested in 1989 engaged in this behaviour regularly, and 7 per cent report having occasionally engaged in this practice (Rosenthal *et al.* 1990). Anal sex was reported as occurring often with regular and casual partners by 7 and 3 per cent respectively of these respondents. In a five-year cross-sectional follow up study of similarly aged university students, the anal sex rates had increased significantly to 5 per cent with casual partners, while remaining at 7 per cent with regular partners (Rosenthal *et al.* 1996b).

An even higher frequency of anal activity among the 16- to 20-year-old group was reported in a British study (Breakwell and Fife-Schaw 1992). Heterosexual anal activity was reported by 9 per cent of boys and girls. Johnson *et al.* (1994) indicate that for their 16- to 59-year-old sample, the highest prevalence of recent anal intercourse occurred among 16- to 24-year-olds who had already experienced vaginal intercourse. Of Turtle *et al.*'s (1989) university students, 8 per cent had engaged in anal sex. Anal intercourse rates are much higher in particular sub-groups. In their study of 16-year-olds, Rosenthal *et al.* (1994) found that 25 per cent of homeless girls and boys reported that they engaged in anal sex with casual or regular partners (or both). Of the homeless young people surveyed by Lhuede and Moore (1994), 32 per cent had engaged in anal intercourse with a regular partner, and 25 per cent with a casual partner. There was little difference between the anal intercourse rates of homeless girls and boys in either study.

The practice of withdrawal of the penis before ejaculation during vaginal intercourse (known as withdrawal) is often not included as a category separate from vaginal intercourse in adolescent sexuality research. Nevertheless it is an important practice to note from the point of view of both pregnancy protection and STD transmission. The belief that withdrawal eliminates risk is mistaken. Even 'successful' withdrawal – less likely among those sexually inexperienced – still carries risk through possible infection carried in the pre-ejaculate or vaginal fluids. Our own studies have indicated that some young people hold the view that withdrawal does not 'count' as an instance of vaginal intercourse. We found among 17- to 20-year-old tertiary students this practice occurred with regular partners for about half the young women and men, and for a substantial minority with casual partners (Rosenthal *et al.* 1990).

Experimentation with homosexuality and bisexuality and the choice of a homosexual identity can occur at any time across the lifespan, but according to Johnson *et al.* (1994), such experimentation and adoption of the gay lifestyle are more likely to occur for men at a relatively young age. They note across their total sample that around 7 per cent of individuals admit attraction to others of the same sex with about 6 per cent of men and 3 per cent of women reporting any homosexual experience ever. Among women who had such experiences, the chances of making a homosexual debut were remarkably consistent at any age from 16 to 59. For men, the chances increased markedly across the teenage and young adult years, after which they remained relatively constant until the late 20s and early 30s, then diminishing rapidly.

Johnson *et al.* (1994), while noting the inadequacy of their data in resolving the issue of stability of sexual orientation, argue nevertheless that earlier homosexual experiences are less likely to lead on to more consistent homosexual behaviour than later ones. Dank (1971) also suggests that later homosexual experiences are more important in predicting persistent homosexual orientation. Interestingly however, Goggin (1993) argues that generally people first define themselves as 'probably' homosexual during the teenage years and that cross-cultural evidence suggests that the more restrictive the culture the later the age at which homosexual self-definition is assumed.

In terms of exclusivity of homosexual behaviour, the Johnson survey showed it to be rare, with the majority of men and women who report having sex with a same-sex partner also having had sex with an opposite-sex partner (over 90 per cent), an estimate rather lower than those reported from purposive or focused samples of homosexual men. What is clear from these data is that experimentation with homosexual practice and to some extent adoption of homosexual or bisexual lifestyles is yet another instance of the variety of sexual activity engaged in during the years of adolescence and youth.

It is noteworthy that sexual practices of young people differ across ethnic groups. An example comes from the study by Rosenthal *et al.* (1990), in which their large sample of 18-year-olds enabled examination of differences among Anglo-Australians and three groups of non-English-speaking background (NESB). Overall, the study found more similarities than differences between the groups, but Greek-Australian boys were the most and Chinese-Australians the least sexually active. There were higher levels of heterosexual anal intercourse reported for Greek-Australians, and boys from this group reported having the most partners and were least likely to view monogamy in a regular relationship as essential for themselves, with only 50 per cent endorsing this view. Of interest was the finding of considerable gender differences in sexual practices of the Greek- and Italian-Australians, but not the Chinese- or Anglo-Australians. The authors caution that their results may underestimate ethnic group differences because the NESB adolescents in their sample were largely ones who had 'succeeded' in the predominantly Anglo-Celtic educational system, and may represent a more acculturated group.

This section has concentrated on what young people *do* sexually, but it is interesting to ponder briefly on sexual beliefs, likes and dislikes, as these too shed light on the diversity of young people's sexual worlds. For example, we asked sexually active single adults (aged 20 to 40 years) recruited in discos and singles bars, 'What aspects of sex do you do for your own pleasure?', and 'What aspects of sex do you do for your partner's pleasure?' (Moore and Rosenthal 1995a). Though many respondents emphasised the mutual aspects of sex, there were clear gender and age differences in inclination. Significantly more women than men cited foreplay as something that they viewed as particularly pleasurable for them and not necessarily their partner, while men had a similar view of receptive oral sex. Younger participants, regardless of sex, were more likely to give oral sex for a partner's pleasure, while anal sex for partner's pleasure was a more common response for older participants. Such diversity underlines the complexities that any safe-sex campaigns must take into account, an issue that is discussed in Chapter 7.

Number of partners

Generally, the majority of the adult population appear conservative with respect to their number of sexual partners. Johnson *et al.* found that, over the last five years, 65 per cent of men and 76 per cent of women from their large sample had had only one sexual partner or none at all. But more detailed analysis reveals what we all suspected, that a substantial minority of individuals change partners frequently. For example 1 per cent of men reported more than twenty-two partners, and 1 per cent of women more than eight partners in the last five years. The possibilities of cross-infection are high among these highly active individuals *and their partners*, especially if condoms are not used. The question is, to what extent is partner changing a feature of adolescent and young adult sexual practice? Is the stereotype of high activity among this age group borne out by the data?

From Johnson *et al.*'s study, the answer is clearly 'yes'. Men and women in the 16 to 24 age group consistently report the greatest numbers of partners, despite this being the group with the highest proportion of respondents who have not yet experienced intercourse. Among this age group, 11 per cent of men and 3 per cent of women reported ten or more heterosexual partners in the last five years. The researchers argue that these figures represent not only an exploration of several relationships before committing to a long-term partnership (which may have also occurred for older age groups when they were in their teens and twenties), but also a genuine generational change in sexual behaviour patterns. They note the difficulties involved in gaining precise estimates of the number of partners that older people had when they were younger, but believe their evidence points to a pattern indicating that individuals now beginning their sex lives will have, on average, a substantially greater number of partners in a lifetime than did their parents.

Our studies indicated that 16 per cent of 18-year-old tertiary student Anglo-Australian males and 8 per cent of similarly aged Anglo-Australian females had had three or more sexual partners in the last six months, although most reported no partners or only one. Subgroups differed markedly however, with 43 per cent of Greek-Australian and 30 per cent of Italian-Australian boys reporting three or more partners over the same period (Rosenthal *et al.* 1990). Outside the tertiary education sector, it is interesting to note somewhat higher rates of sexual activity among 18-year-olds. In a study of unemployed young people, 90.5 per cent had engaged in penetrative sexual activities (Buzwell 1993). Most of these young people had had a sexual partner in the preceding six months, with 19 per cent reporting three or more partners. In a separate study of a younger group, 16-year-old Anglo-Australian, Greek-Australian and homeless young people were questioned about their sexual behaviour and sexual beliefs (Rosenthal *et al.* 1994). The homeless group was significantly more sexually active than the other groups and had more partners. Homeless boys reported an average of twelve partners, and girls an average of seven partners, in the preceding six months, with a maximum exceeding 100 for both sexes, compared with a maximum of five (and an average of between zero and one) for home-based youths. The higher levels of sexual activity of these young people were confirmed in a study of eighty homeless young people aged 15 to 20 years (Lhuede and Moore 1994). Boys in this group were more sexually active than girls.

Beliefs about faithfulness and monogamy

Are you always faithful to your partner?

So far, it depends how far into the relationship you are. If I was interested in someone else I would want to break it off [with the current partner] first. *(16-year-old girl)*

Beliefs about whether you and your partner should be faithful or monogamous in a relationship are relevant to the discussion of safe sex, because if you are both uninfected and both stay faithful, there is no problem. But partners can misunderstand each other's expectations and beliefs, or intentions can be misrepresented, or not carried out. In these cases, infection becomes a clear possibility, and one that poses not only a threat to health but to emotional well-being because of the perceived breach of trust.

Research in this area is informative. Among the 16-year-olds interviewed by Buzwell *et al.* (1992), only about 40 per cent said that they are (or would be) always faithful to their sexual partner. There were differences between subgroups, however, in that 97 per cent of Greek-Australian girls indicated their intent to be totally faithful, in comparison, for example, with only 40 per cent of Anglo-Australian girls. Significant numbers of the latter group said they were usually faithful and/or tried to be but were not always successful, and 12 per cent said they would only be faithful in a long-term relationship. This 'regular–casual' distinction was also made quite strongly by Greek-Australian boys, 20 per cent of whom would only be faithful if they were in a long-term partnership. Rosenthal and Moore's (1991) older adolescents were similarly not totally committed to monogamy. In this study, young people were asked if they would be faithful to their partner in *a long-term relationship* and if they expected faithfulness in return. Most girls believed they would be and expected likewise of their partners (95 per cent in both cases). While most boys (86 per cent) expected their female partner to be monogamous, only three-quarters had the same expectation of themselves. An example illustrates the point:

Are you always faithful to your partner?

I don't think I would be because you know she will be there and that she thinks a lot of you. And if there is an opportunity for, say, a one-night stand, and you like her in a physical sort of way, then I reckon most guys would be unfaithful. Because if they think they won't get caught, they know nothing will happen to their relationship.

The norm for young people is that of 'serial monogamy', incorporating the idea of mutual faithfulness and commitment to the current partner as if he or she were to be permanent. In reality, the serial nature of relationships often describes them more adequately than the monogamy aspect, which is not consistently upheld. Young people, beginning their sexual lives earlier than their parents and marrying later, are likely to have more partners in a lifetime than was the norm in previous generations. Further, the many exceptions to patterns of lifetime monogamy or conservative serial monogamy increase markedly the possibilities of STD transmission if safe practices are not consistently used. The extent of uptake of these practices is discussed in the following section.

UNSAFE SEX

As DiClemente (1993b) points out, although sexual abstinence is clearly the most effective strategy for prevention of sexually transmitted disease, it is not realistic to expect that many adolescents will adopt this strategy, especially once sexual activity has begun. As we have seen, most young people begin their sexual careers in the late teenage years, engage in a wider variety of sexual practices than did their parents, and are highly likely to have more than one partner over a lifetime. But critical to an assessment of the risk of sexual disease faced by these young people is knowledge of the extent to which their sexual practices are 'safe'. Most importantly, this relates to whether, in penetrative sex, condoms are used consistently, and discussion of this issue is the major focus of this section. Other risk factors, less common but of serious impact to particular groups, are also discussed, namely intravenous (IV) drug use, and the increased STD risk among specific sub-groups of sexually active young people of poor health status, such as the homeless. Analysis of adolescents' beliefs about their level of risk and discussion of the predominant mythologies that serve to limit the uptake of safe practice occurs in the following chapters.

Non-use of condoms

Some comments about condoms from a group of 16-year-old girls illustrate the ambiguous feelings young people have about them.

How do you feel about condoms?

I don't really like them, they're annoying – getting rid of them after you have finished, and putting them on.

They are great, they are good, but they are annoying. They're really good not just for pregnancy but for diseases.

I think they are fine, but it can be worrying if it breaks, there can be a bit of stress on that.

They are not bad, I prefer not to use them, but I guess you have to.

Although there has been a considerable increase in young people's acceptance of condoms over the past decade, studies of condom *use* show that many young people use them inconsistently or not at all. The increase in condom use rates appears to have occurred largely because most young people now use condoms 'sometimes'. The meaning of this is complex from the point of view of adolescent sexual health. On the positive side it indicates increased exposure to condoms and the potential for improved skill in negotiating their use, at both interpersonal and purely mechanical levels. On the other hand, it indicates that protection is not consistent. Young people are in fact (a) being influenced by situational factors within sexual encounters, such as high arousal, alcohol and drug use, or partner reluctance, or (b) making judgements about particular partners and/ or sexual situations that lead them to reject the need to use condoms. Examples of partner judgements are that 'this partner is too nice to be diseased', or 'this partner is someone I love therefore must be safe'. Examples of situational judgements are those based on the notion that bodily fluids are not going to be exchanged in this sexual situation, or if they are, it will still be safe because the activity is unlikely to lead to HIV infection. Discussion of each of these factors occurs in more detail in Chapters 4 and 5. The problem is that while young people in many Western countries have so far 'got away with' using these flawed types of judgements and escaped HIV infection, as the infection rates increase in the population their luck could run out. The same is true for infection with many other STDs, and for some of these the number of infections could increase at an even greater rate than is potentially possible for HIV. Details of research concerning adolescent condom use follows.

Hingson and Strunin (1992) surveyed HIV/AIDS knowledge, attitudes, beliefs and behaviours of adolescents in Massachusetts, USA, in 1986, 1988 and 1990. They used state-wide random digit-dial telephone surveys, yielding 16- to 19-year-old samples of 826, 1,762, and 1,152 respectively. While the number of young people who adopted condom use specifically because of the AIDS epidemic rose markedly over the five years of the study, by 1990 still only 37 per cent of sexually active young people were using condoms consistently. Further, the proportion of the age group who were sexually active had increased by 10 per cent from 55 per cent in 1986 to 65 per cent in 1990. Consequently the percentage of the later cohorts having unprotected intercourse was not much lower than the percentage in 1986, despite increases in knowledge, educational campaigns and wide publicity.

In Britain, Johnson *et al.* defined unsafe heterosex as having had two or more heterosexual partners in the last year and never having used a condom. These authors recognised that this definition underestimates risky behaviour, for example having one partner who is unfaithful, or using condoms only sometimes. Using this stringent definition, their data showed that the likelihood of unsafe sex decreases with age, with men under 25 at most risk. Also in Britain, Breakwell and Fife-Schaw's (1992) review of the literature came to apparently different conclusions, indicating that condom use declined with age. However, their sample was of young people only, aged 16 to 25. The age decline in safe-sex practice was attributed to older sexually active individuals in the youth age group more likely to have established stable monogamous relationships. Also Breakwell and Fife-Schaw used a different definition of unsafe sex, counting all non-condom use as unsafe, independent of number of partners. Their review underscores some of the methodological difficulties in comparing unsafe sex rates among young people. Across the seven British studies they reviewed (published between 1987 and 1992), the number of non-virgins using a condom in their most recent sexual encounter varied between 15 and 66 per cent, a variation that was partly but not entirely due to the different age subgroups studied within the 16- to 25-year range.

In Australia, condom use has been investigated in a number of studies of school-aged teenagers (Centre for Adolescent Health 1992; Dunne *et al.* 1993a; Howard 1991; Rosenthal *et al.* 1994; Weisberg *et al.* 1992). In a national survey of high-school students, Dunne and his colleagues found that boys were more likely than girls to report that a condom was always used when they had sex: 53, 46 and 45 per cent of the boys and 32, 37 and 24 per cent of the girls in years 10, 11 and 12 respectively claimed that they never had sex *without* a condom. However, 12, 9 and 12 per cent of non-virgin boys and 17, 7 and 12 per cent of girls, in years 10, 11 and 12 respectively, reported that they never had sex *with* a condom. Thus a large percentage of both boys and girls fitted the 'sometimes' category in their response to condom use. Almost half the girls and about 30 per cent of the boys in each year reported that they did not use a condom the last time that they had sex. The most common reason for girls' failure to use condoms was that they were on the contraceptive pill. Several other common reasons were cause for alarm. These included trust in their partner (19 per cent) and perceived low risk – 'clean partner' (15 per cent). In only 8 per cent of cases, the reason offered was that both partners had been tested for HIV/STDs. Responses by boys followed a similar pattern of inappropriate reasons, in terms of protection against HIV/STDs.

Among samples of post-secondary young Australians, research has repeatedly found low and inconsistent condom use (Gallois *et al.* 1992a; Lhuede and Moore 1994; Rosenthal *et al.* 1990; Turtle *et al.* 1989). For example, in the Rosenthal study, it was found that only about one-third of those students who had previously had intercourse with a casual partner always used a condom, and only one-fifth always used a condom with a regular (steady) partner. Of concern was the finding that a small but significant number of students had taken part in anal sex with a regular or casual partner without using a condom, a finding in line with that of Breakwell and Fife-Schaw (1991) in Britain.

There are also disturbing numbers of adolescents engaging in sex with more than one partner without using a condom (Rosenthal *et al.* 1990). However, it is important to note that while young people do have multiple partners, they continue to make a distinction between casual and regular partners, and there is evidence to suggest that sexual practices are modified accordingly. Overall, young people engage in less risky behaviours with casual partners than with regular partners. In particular, young women are more likely to use a condom if the sexual encounter is casual or does not occur 'in a relationship' (Abbott 1988; Crawford *et al.* 1990; Rosenthal and Moore 1991; Wyn 1993). For example, Abbott's study of adolescent girls in Canberra showed that 55 per cent believed that having sex only with a steady boyfriend was a safe-sex option, and this was the main change they had made to protect themselves. However, it is a concern that only a very short time span need elapse before a relationship is considered regular and that such an indiscriminate, flexible transition point may determine young women's use of condoms. For example, if adolescents think that the safe-sex message pertains only to casual relationships, yet consider a partner to be regular after only six months (and, in some cases, after as short a period as a week) then they may not heed safe-sex messages.

Intravenous drug use

Even lower levels of condom use are reported among young intravenous drug users (IDUs) (Louie *et al.* 1996); thus this group faces the 'double jeopardy' of possible infection through sexual or drug-related risk behaviours. Only 12 per cent of this sample always used a condom with a regular partner, and only 22 per cent with a casual partner. There was a large gender difference, with girls reporting higher condom use (41 per cent) than boys (14 per cent). Almost half never used a condom with a regular partner and 21 per cent never did so with a casual partner. This low condom use for IDUs is consistent with findings of another small Australian study (Loxley and Ovenden 1992) and is especially worrying among a group already at risk.

A Glasgow-based study of non clinic-based intravenous drug users involved interviews with these individuals while they were purchasing injecting equipment in a retail pharmacy (McKeganey and Barnard 1990). The population was generally young (mean age 23 for the women and 25 for the men), with most respondents reporting starting injecting when they were 16 or 17 years of age. Sharing of injecting equipment was common, especially between sexual partners. Many of those who rejected sharing as a general habit said they might ask to borrow another's equipment if they were badly in need of a hit and unable to procure their own equipment readily. The majority of drug injectors in this sample were unaware of their actual HIV status and were not using any form of barrier contraception. An apparent lack of knowledge about their risk of transmitting HIV to sexual partners was exhibited. The belief seemed to be that if you were in a steady relationship, or knew your partner well enough, infection would not occur. The possibility that these IDUs might *transmit* the disease to their partners did not seem to be understood. Klee's (1990) study of IDUs in north-west England at around the same time showed similar results. Seventy-five per cent of the sexually active IDUs in her sample never used condoms, and many of these expressed no intention to change to safer sexual practices.

Vulnerable groups

Sondheimer (1992) notes that homeless youths are at extremely high risk for acquiring HIV and for experiencing early illness and death. Evidence concerning their multiple risk factors, along with those of other highly vulnerable groups, will be discussed in this section.

Among a homeless group of youths in Australia, Lhuede and Moore (1994) showed that nearly half had used IV drugs, most were sexually active, and of these 70 per cent never or only sometimes used condoms. Added to the danger of this lethal combination of risk factors was the information that sharing needles was a frequent practice and needle cleaning did not always follow approved methods. King *et al.* (1989) drew similar conclusions from a nationwide study of Canadian youth. A further risk factor among these homeless young people arose from their lack of knowledge of their sexual partners' drug and sexual histories. Nearly half the females and a quarter of the males said they had had a sexual partner who used IV drugs, and many were uncertain of past partners' drug-taking status. It is well known that young people who experience the vulnerable lifestyle of life on the streets are more prone to a range of illnesses and infections, and this, too, may predispose these young people to sexually transmitted infections. A further point is that prostitution can become an economic reality for homeless girls and boys, providing money for food, shelter, drugs and clothing. Hersch (1988) suggests that American homeless youths who sell sex are less likely to take precautions, providing the following quotation:

> they [clients] want fantasies, condoms aren't part of fantasies.
> AIDS isn't part of fantasies.
> (young female prostitute quoted in Hersch 1988: 29)

Sondheimer (1992), in summarising US studies, argues that sexual activity with multiple partners is the major risk factor for homeless adolescents, rather than IV drug use. But she notes that drug use, particularly crack, 'is a key cause for concern because it provides an impetus for engaging in prostitution and having multiple sex partners' (1992: 75). This high risk level does not seem to arise from a lack of information, with King *et al.*'s (1989) study indicating that often street youths were more knowledgeable about AIDS than college students. The uncertainties of life on the street and the histories of those who choose or are coerced or forced into this lifestyle provide more persuasive forces against safe sex than simply 'knowing better'.

Incarcerated youths too are at high risk of infection with HIV and other STDs (Morris *et al.* 1992). Surveys conducted in 1989 and 1990 by these researchers indicated low overall prevalence of condom use (both inside and outside prison), with 65 per cent and 67 per cent respectively never using condoms and only 7 and 4 per cent respectively consistently using them. Possibilities for cross-infection in prison are very high, not only because of unsafe sex and drug practices, but because so many of these young people already have STD infections. For example, in Los Angeles, 45 to 50 per cent of females entering juvenile detention centres had an STD (Brady *et al.* 1988). The rate was lower for males (15 to 20 per cent), but other surveys suggest much higher rates for incarcerated homosexual, bisexual and black male youth (Morris *et al.* 1992). (Corresponding data for females are unavailable.) An issue to be dealt with in prisons is clearly the ready supply of condoms, a difficult one as sex is a prohibited activity. But there is no doubt that it occurs. Further, the relatively short stays in prison for most incarcerated youths, their bad habits in terms of safe sex and their propensity for multiple partnering make this group an infection 'time bomb', unless appropriate education strategies can lead to changes in practice.

Groups of young people with high rates of infection already, who interact with each other sexually, are of course at the highest level of risk. Therefore homosexual men in areas such as New York and San Francisco are extremely vulnerable to HIV infection if they do not use condoms. This is not because their sexual practices *per se* are any more risky than those of, say, heterosexuals in Brighton or Vancouver, but because the chances of having sex with an infected partner are greater. This is not always clearly understood, by young people or adults. An outcome of the misunderstanding is a sense of safety about unprotected heterosexual practice that would be misplaced if infection rates in the heterosexual population began to rise, as is the case in sub-Saharan Africa and parts of Asia.

SEX, LIES, AND RISK OF INFECTION

One strategy apparently used quite frequently by young people to avoid HIV risk is to endeavour to select partners whom they judge to be of low risk of already being infected. The myth that 'you can tell by looking' will be discussed further in Chapter 5. What is of interest here is the advice given in some public health forums to facilitate AIDS prevention through discussing with potential partners your own and your partner's past sexual and IV drug history, then negotiating safer sexual practices (Cline *et al.* 1992). To conduct such discussions clearly involves skills and confidence not always present among the young. In fact, Cline *et al.*'s study of over 500 US college students indicated that only about 6 per cent of the heterosexual and sexually experienced students had talked to partners about condom use, although about two-thirds had discussed AIDS in a more general way. Some quotations from our own study of 16-year-olds indicates some of the problems faced by young people in broaching topics such as infection status and past history of HIV risk behaviour.

Do you ask them [about STDs] before you sleep with them?

I guess it would be embarrassing. It's not the sort of question you ask, but you would think about it probably.

No, I don't think it is necessary. I would fish for it like asking about previous relationships. But I wouldn't want to put her on the spot like that.

No, I don't think so. I don't know. If you had an inclination, you would probe a bit deeper and ask them casually.

No, I haven't, because most of the guys I've slept with I have known pretty much all about them because I've known them for ages.

Most worrying is the finding of Cochran and Mays (1990) who showed that even when young people do engage in past-history discussions, the information they gain may not always be truthful. Among unmarried college students, 34 per cent of the men admitted having lied in order to have sex. Further, 47 per cent of the men and 42 per cent of the women said they would tell new partners that they had had fewer past sexual partners than was actually the case. In addition, 22 per cent of the men and 10 per cent of the women would not disclose the existence of another partner to a new partner, and over one-third of both sexes would not admit to their partner if they had been unfaithful. These researchers note that 'dishonesty is an intimate feature of dating life' (Mays and Cochran 1993: 86). Disclosure of past drug use, homosexual encounters, or a large number of (or even any) past sexual partners may jeopardise a new relationship, be highly embarrassing, or influence the future of the relationship in unwished-for ways (Derelega and Chaikin 1975). The non-use of condoms among young people becomes even more a cause for concern when viewed in this context.

CONCLUSIONS

There are several themes that arise from the research outlined above, and these provide the background information necessary for any understanding of young people's sexual behaviour. First, adolescence has frequently been portrayed as a period of sexual experimentation. While this is not true of all adolescents, there is certainly a pattern of sexual liberalism that involves high levels of premarital sex, casual sex, and multiple partnering. Second, the number of young people who use condoms every time they have sex is extremely low. Third, although intravenous drug use is uncommon, those who engage in it frequently share needles, use inappropriate cleaning techniques, and/or have unprotected sex. Sub-groups of young people such as the homeless often engage in all the above behaviours, and this places them at particularly serious risk. Finally, young people do not always truthfully represent their past sexual histories to new partners. So what we have among the youth of Western nations is the potential for HIV and other STD rates to rise, quite markedly in some sub-groups, unless behaviour change does not ensue. Techniques for promoting such behaviour change are discussed in Chapter 7.

3 Understanding the risk

Young people's knowledge of and attitudes towards STDs

KNOWLEDGE OF HIV/AIDS

In early research, a key assumption was that unsafe sexual behaviour stemmed from a lack of knowledge about the transmission of HIV. So if young people knew the consequences of unsafe sexual behaviour then they would not engage in such behaviours. Although early US studies of adolescent knowledge of HIV/AIDS transmission (DiClemente *et al.* 1986; Strunin and Hingson 1987) reported that large numbers of young people had an inaccurate understanding of the way in which HIV is transmitted, by the late 1980s and early 1990s the majority of American youths seemed to have learned the lessons about HIV transmission (e.g. Bowler *et al.* 1992; Boyer and Kegeles 1991; Sonenstein *et al.* 1989). Most misconceptions had disappeared, although some persisted, such as the belief that HIV can be acquired through donating blood (Andre and Bormann 1991). Unfortunately, inadequate knowledge was most apparent among young people who belonged to high-risk groups such as delinquent youths and school drop-outs (Hingson and Strunin 1992; Rotheram-Borus *et al.* 1991). In several studies, African-Americans and Latinos were also found to be less knowledgeable than white Americans (e.g. Bell *et al.* 1990; DiClemente *et al.* 1988).

Like their American peers, Australian youths appear to be knowledgeable about HIV/AIDS and this knowledge has increased over time. Compared to an early survey in 1986–7, which showed that only 56 per cent of young Australian people aged 16 to 24 were 'knowledgeable' about AIDS (Commonwealth Department of Community Services and Health 1988), most recent studies (Crawford *et al.* 1990, 1994; Dunne *et al.* 1993a; Rosenthal *et al.* 1990; Turtle *et al.* 1989) have shown adolescents to have high levels of knowledge about HIV transmission and AIDS.

There is evidence of uneven knowledge among specific groups of young people. Consistent with reports from the United States, in which foreign-born students were significantly less likely to know the major modes of HIV transmission than non-immigrants (Hingson *et al.* 1991), Australian youths from non-English-speaking backgrounds, and especially young women, had lower levels of knowledge than their Anglo-Celtic peers (Rosenthal *et al.* 1990). There is also some evidence that homeless youths and those from rural areas have less accurate knowledge about risky behaviour than their home-based or urban peers (Matthews *et al.* 1990).

Other Australian studies have uncovered general gaps in young people's knowledge about HIV. Young people have clear information about the ways in which HIV is transmitted, yet there seems to be uncertainty regarding the circumstances by which HIV is *not* transmitted (Gallois *et al.* 1992b). Many college students were uncertain about the risks associated with oral sex, deep kissing and withdrawal and some falsely believed that mutual masturbation is unsafe with a casual partner, but that unprotected vaginal intercourse is safe with a regular partner (Crawford *et al.* 1990; Turtle *et al.* 1989). Dunne and his colleagues (1993a) also reported some inconsistencies in high-school students' knowledge. For example, a large minority was uncertain about some specific facts, such as whether a person could get HIV from mosquitoes, a finding reported elsewhere (McCamish 1992). Although the role of blood in the transmission of HIV appears to be consistently understood, a substantial minority of young people are unaware that HIV could be transmitted through vaginal fluids, and many do not distinguish between disease prevention and contraception, believing that condoms are unnecessary if other methods of contraception are being used (Greig and Raphael 1989; Orr *et al.* 1992; Wyn and Stewart 1991).

DOES KNOWLEDGE EQUAL SAFE SEX?

In spite of high levels of knowledge, young people do not appear to be applying that knowledge to their sexual behaviour. A number of studies, both in Australia and in other countries, have shown that higher levels of knowledge are unrelated to safe-sex practices (Boldero *et al.* 1992; Kegeles *et al.* 1988; Keller *et al.* 1988; Richard and van der Pligt 1991; Weissman *et al.* 1989). An American study of adolescents over one year (Kegeles *et al.* 1988) found that knowing that condoms prevented HIV transmission did not lead to a greater intention to use condoms, nor an increase in actual condom use.

Similarly, in their sample of Australian tertiary students, Turtle *et al.* (1989) reported a marked discrepancy between beliefs about engaging in safe sex and actually doing so. Studies examining the relationship between knowledge and behaviour in high-risk groups have found the same inconsistencies. Two American studies reported high rates of HIV risk behaviours among runaways (Rotheram-Borus and Koopman 1991) and incarcerated adolescents (DiClemente *et al.* 1991), despite moderately high levels of AIDS knowledge in these groups. The findings of these studies clearly indicate that knowledge is not necessarily directly linked with behaviour change.

WHAT IS 'KNOWLEDGE'?

The lack of a relationship between knowledge and behaviour has led some researchers to question the nature of the knowledge that young people have about HIV/AIDS. It has been argued that a distinction needs to be made between 'factual knowledge' and 'understanding', and care must be taken not to infer automatically that high levels of factual knowledge reflect a thorough understanding of an issue (Rosenthal *et al.* 1996c). In a sample of young teenagers, Slattery (1991) found that, while a large majority (90 per cent) knew that sexual behaviour is associated with HIV transmission, and many (68 per cent) knew of the risks of contact with blood, most of these adolescents showed minimal or no understanding of the exact nature of the danger. For instance, many of these young people believed that contact with menstrual blood was more likely to give a person HIV than blood from a leg wound. Slattery concluded that while some young people had specific factual knowledge about HIV/AIDS, only half of them displayed acceptable levels of understanding and accurate knowledge.

A similar conclusion is drawn from a study by Rosenthal *et al.* (1996c). Knowledge levels assessed using a standard self-report questionnaire were high, even among the youngest group studied (10-year-olds), consistent with earlier findings. However, most of the younger and many of the older respondents, when interviewed about their 'knowledge', revealed limited understanding of HIV/AIDS, often in spite of high scores on the questionnaire (from which high levels of 'knowledge' might be inferred). The following extracts from two 15-year-olds' interviews demonstrate this point well. Both had high scores on the 'true–false' questionnaire, but it is clear that their understanding of HIV/AIDS differed considerably.

How does someone get AIDS? The two most common ways of getting AIDS are through unprotected sex and sharing needles. But the person may not get AIDS; they might just become a carrier of the HIV virus. *How does unprotected sex cause AIDS?* If a man does not wear a condom he can pass the virus through his semen or get it from the woman's fluids. *How would you know if he had AIDS?* I wouldn't know for a long time. *Why is that?* Well, the symptoms of AIDS do not show up for years because there is a long incubation period. *What do you mean by symptoms?* The person actually catches other viruses and diseases more easily because AIDS has affected their immunity. *What happens during the incubation period?* The AIDS virus kills off the immune system.

How does someone get AIDS? By having sex *(said in a tentative manner). How does having sex cause AIDS?* It's from the blood or something. *Can you tell me anything more?* It just goes through the. organs. *Would you know if someone had AIDS?* Yes, I think I would. *Can you explain to me why you think you would know?* They would look really sick. *Don't they lose their hair or something? (Pause)* I think they can get rashes as well.

(Rosenthal *et al.* 1996c: 518)

Across all ages, understanding conformed to a developmental pattern that was consistent with these young people's cognitive level and with research on understanding of other illnesses (Glaun 1991). Glaun found that children's and adolescents' understanding of illness accorded with a shift from 'novice' to 'expert' and could be characterised as a progression of increasing cognitive complexity along a variety of dimensions relating to cause, prevention and cure. Applying this model to HIV/AIDS, Rosenthal *et al.* (1996c) were able to map increasingly complex thinking about the disease, for example in the nature of the causal factors – from a single unitary causal explanation ('You get it from bad blood') to the naming of multiple factors, with some routes of infection being more common than others.

It is probably more likely to be caused by having unprotected sex with someone who has the AIDS virus, but it can also be contracted by sharing needles, and pregnant mothers can even pass it on to their baby. You can also get it from a blood transfusion even though it is less likely.

(Rosenthal *et al.* 1996c: 511)

Another dimension that revealed increasing complexity was related to the temporal relationship between the perceived cause and onset of AIDS. Children's thinking at the least complex level identifies causal events in the immediate environment that just precede onset of illness ('You stand next to someone who's got it and then you've got it'). At the most complex level, there is recognition of a delay between cause and effect and acknowledgement that AIDS is an illness that has different stages.

> The incubation period is about six months when the AIDS virus attacks and takes over the antibodies. Then it can take two to ten years before the onset of external symptoms.
>
> (Rosenthal *et al.* 1996c: 511)

The findings of these studies suggest that understanding about HIV/AIDS develops in line with children's and adolescents' cognitive capacity, and that many young people do not have a high level of understanding of HIV/AIDS, although they may have an adequate grasp of the relevant facts. This absence of genuine understanding may, in part, explain the reported lack of association between knowledge and behaviour change.

KNOWLEDGE OF STDs

Almost nothing is known about young people's understanding of STDs other than HIV/AIDS, despite the significant health threat that STDs pose. This lack of research is only now being addressed. In the national study of Australian high-school students conducted by Dunne and his colleagues, the high levels of knowledge about HIV transmission were not matched by knowledge of other STDs. While the most commonly named STD was herpes, less than half of year 12 (17-year-old) students and less than one-third of year 11 (16-year-old) students named this disease. Syphilis, now extremely uncommon, was named by one-third of year 12 students, but chlamydia, currently an STD of considerable concern, was named by only 5 per cent of year 12 boys and 19 per cent of girls. Fewer than half of the respondents could name three or more symptoms of STDs. Analogous findings were reported in a recent study that examined the knowledge of STDs in a large sample of Victorian high-school students (Smith *et al.* 1995) and in other studies, both in Australia (Wright *et al.* 1991; Wyn 1993; Wyn and Stewart 1991) and the United States (Benton *et al.* 1993).

Equally low levels of knowledge about STDs other than HIV/AIDS have been found among older students (Minichiello *et al.* 1994;

Rosenthal and Moore 1994). Almost all the young people in Rosenthal and Moore's study had heard of HIV/AIDS, yet a large number had *not* heard of the other listed STDs: chlamydia (66 per cent), gonorrhoea (42 per cent), herpes (30 per cent), and genital warts/HPV (32 per cent). Of those young people who had heard of the other STDs, a large minority believed that these STDs were either 'not very' or 'not at all' serious, and did not have long-term consequences. Many respondents were uncertain of their own or others' ability to know if they had a particular STD and had very poor understanding of the causes of these STDs.

As with HIV/AIDS, there are differences in young people's knowledge of STDs. Girls on the whole are more knowledgeable than boys and, predictably, older students have greater knowledge than those who are younger. There is some evidence that children of non-English-speaking immigrants have poorer knowledge (Dunne *et al.* 1993b; Minichiello *et al.* 1994).

What can we conclude about young people's knowledge? Knowledge about HIV/AIDS is encouragingly high among most young people, suggesting that information campaigns designed to increase knowledge have been effective. However, knowledge about HIV/AIDS appears to be necessary but not sufficient for preventive action. On the other hand, young people are alarmingly ignorant about STDs. The advent of HIV/AIDS as a serious threat to young people and the community at large has resulted in considerable resources being devoted to educating people about a single STD. While other STDs do not have such uniformly adverse outcomes as HIV, their greater incidence, prevalence and consequent morbidity among adolescents and young adults require that more resources be devoted to addressing the educational needs of young people in this respect. An increase in knowledge about the more prevalent STDs among young people is likely to increase their perception of risk as a result of knowing an infected person. This may then result in safer behaviour, which has the positive side-effect of decreasing the risk of HIV.

HOW IS KNOWLEDGE ABOUT HIV AND OTHER STDs GAINED?

Sources of information

We know that the perceived attitudes and values of significant others have an important shaping effect on an individual's intention to act in a particular manner and, ultimately, on the performance of that action

(Ajzen and Fishbein 1977; Ajzen and Madden 1986). Among adolescents, two such key influences are parents and peers. Surprisingly, the impact of these two developmentally significant groups on young people's sexual practices has not been a major focus of interest among researchers. Older students and high-school students describe their parents as non-liberal in their sexual attitudes and unlikely to discuss sex or safe sex with them, especially compared with peers (Dunne *et al.* 1993a; Moore and Rosenthal 1991a; Stancombe 1994; Wright *et al.* 1991). Lack of confidence in talking to parents about sex is one reason cited for the communication gap, but girls were more confident than boys. Young people also claim to feel more confident that they could talk to parents about the specific issues of HIV and other STDs than about sex more generally.

Parents' points of view on the communication process are rarely invited. In one study of the parental perspective, parents regarded themselves as being highly influential, relative to other information sources, on the knowledge and practices of their own 16-year-old son or daughter (Rosenthal and Collis 1996). While almost all parents believed that they were open to discussions about sex, only 66 per cent reported that they had actually discussed sexual matters with their teenage son or daughter. Ironically, all the parents questioned had an idealised view of their own teenager, and their relationship with him or her. Compared with other parents' teenagers, their own teenager was rated as less sexually active, more responsible about using condoms, more confident about sexual matters, more communicative with parents, and more influenced by parents than by other sources of sexual information. While it might sustain them in their difficult role as parents of a teenager to believe that they are doing a good job, especially in the sexual arena, this rosy glow needs to be carefully interpreted. In the context of little discussion about sex between parents and adolescents, we need to ask how parents' judgements are being made. We need, also, to consider the barriers to parent–adolescent communication about this private and often taboo subject, and these are discussed in Chapter 7.

While the influence of parents and peers is constantly addressed in textbooks on adolescent development, in this information-rich environment and in the realm of sexuality especially, there are many other potential sources of information and influence. Young people are constantly exposed to large amounts of information through the mass media, and educational institutions, among other sources. The information is of varying quality and relevance and requires them to decide which sources they should believe and trust, and how to use this information. The sources available for young people to gain information about STDs include school programmes or teachers, the mass media, and health professionals. While there are many options available to young people for accessing information, the role of the media in providing a substantial amount of information to young people about health issues (and specifically STDs and sexual matters) is demonstrated in a number of studies in the United States and Great Britain (Abraham *et al.* 1991; Andre and Bormann 1991; Bell *et al.* 1990; Harris *et al.* 1991) and in Australia (Rosenthal and Smith 1994; Slattery 1991; Stancombe 1994; Wilders and MacCallum 1990; Wyn 1993).

The power of the media can be summed up in the large number of 'Dear Doctor' columns in magazines read avidly by young girls and in the frankness of the questions addressed to these 'experts'. The following sample from just one Australian publication popular with young teenagers reveals a touching faith in the doctor's ability to diagnose and cure through the pages of the magazine.

Is it true that you can catch an STD from just kissing?

Two years ago I had a lot of warts removed. Could I catch genital warts by inserting a tampon with the same finger I had warts on?

I'm a 13-year-old boy and I have a problem. For about 3 weeks I've been getting this clear, jelly-like stuff in my jocks and after that I get blood coming out of my penis. Am I having periods? Am I turning into a girl?

I'm 16 and on the pill. When my boyfriend and I have sex, a white discharge comes out afterwards. Is something wrong, or is this normal?

Source credibility

We know from a large body of research on effective communication that the credibility of a source is an important factor affecting the persuasiveness of a communication. Sources that are highly credible are more effective at changing attitudes and beliefs and even behaviours than their less credible counterparts. Both the expertise of the source and the perceived trustworthiness of that source are important aspects of credibility. So if we are to look at the sources of young people's information about STDs, including HIV/AIDS, and their impact on beliefs and behaviours, we need also to take account of whether young people regard those sources as credible and thus persuasive.

It seems that young people of both sexes want to receive information from booklets, and school-based health education programmes, although girls still prefer to acquire information from books or magazines (Rosenthal and Smith 1994). Health professionals, especially doctors, are high on the list of preferred sources of information about STDs, but young people report that they rarely use these sources (Abraham *et al.* 1991; Dunne *et al.* 1993a; Rosenthal and Smith 1994). One study reports that a large majority of their high-school students would seek advice from the medical profession if they actually had symptoms or evidence of an infection with an STD, but very few would consult a health professional for preventive advice (Wright *et al.* 1991).

The most trusted sources of information are those perceived as having 'legitimate' knowledge, such as health professionals and school sources. The finding that doctors are trusted sources of information who are rarely used points to the need to integrate health professionals into the education strategies used for young people. The difficulty with this approach is that high trust in these sources is not matched by equally high preference for seeking them out. Paradoxically, the mass media, although the most common source of information used by most students, lack credibility and are not preferred as a source.

Clearly, frequent use of a particular information source should not be regarded as an indication that this source is effective. There is a need to make accessible to young people those sources that they prefer and trust and those that are seen to have legitimate knowledge. Why are some highly trusted sources such as health professionals *not* used and unlikely to be accessed? There are many reasons why young people do not seek information from health professionals. These include the high cost of consultations, concern that moral judgements would be made about them, doubts about confidentiality with particular fears that information would reach parents, the perceived disease orientation of doctors and feelings of doubt as to their ability to broach such a sensitive topic with a doctor.

One potential avenue of providing readily available trusted sources is to extend the use of health professionals by commonly used media. For example, anecdotal evidence does suggest that advice columns in magazines written by doctors do have an impact on young girls, as do radio talk-back programmes with doctors. Another strategy, given the importance of peer influence, is to combine educator legitimacy with peer status. One such strategy currently being used is to have medical students return to their former schools to teach students about HIV and other STDs (Short 1993). These young educators, only a few years older than their audience of high-school students, having acquired the necessary knowledge through their medical studies, have legitimacy conferred through their status as 'young doctors' (or doctors-to-be).

While we must be careful that the education programmes provided by these sorts of informants are informed by best education practice, there is certainly the potential for maximising acceptance of messages by using legitimate and preferred sources of information. A further complicating factor, though, is that some groups of young people are restricted in the sources of information that they can access. For example, homeless youths may have limited access to education as well as other media sources and are unlikely to have parents or siblings who can provide them with information. For these young people, youth workers may represent the best and most appropriate sources of information (Matthews *et al.* 1990).

DETERMINING RISK

Perceptions of risk

Young people's behaviour is commonly regarded as being determined, at least in part, by the belief that they are invulnerable to the hazards that befall other individuals. This perceived sense of personal invulnerability to risk is of particular relevance to the study of young people's sexual risk taking. The extent to which young people misperceive their risk of contracting HIV and other STDs and the relationship between risk perception and risky practices are important in planning effective intervention strategies. We know that the sexual practices of many young people place themselves and their partners at risk of STDs, including HIV. The question arises as to whether young people engage in these practices in spite of recognising their risky nature or whether they perceive, rightly or wrongly, that their risk of infection is low.

Unlike their gay peers, few heterosexual young people believe that HIV/AIDS is an issue relevant to their own lives. Most believe that their risk of being infected with HIV/AIDS is low (e.g. Abrams *et al.* 1990; Crawford *et al.* 1990; Gallois *et al.* 1990; McCamish 1992; Moore and Rosenthal 1991b; Wright 1990). Even among homeless young people, many of whom are engaging in high-risk behaviours, there is a disturbingly low level of perceived risk of HIV/AIDS (Lhuede and Moore 1994; Matthews *et al.* 1990).

The risk of being infected with other STDs is likewise perceived to be low (Lucke *et al.* 1993; Moore and Rosenthal 1995b). In a nation-wide survey of young Australians, aged 14 to 24 (Australian Broadcasting Commission 1993), young men and women believed that they were unlikely to contract an STD, including HIV/AIDS. For each disease (including gonorrhoea, syphilis, chlamydia, HIV/AIDS, genital warts, herpes), between 85 and 91 per cent of the respondents felt that they were 'not likely' to contract this disease. Among the high-school students studied by Lucke and colleagues the main reasons given for low perceptions of risk were: not sharing needles/syringes, not injecting drugs, using a condom when having sex, and abstaining from sex. Realistically, sexually experienced adolescents were more likely to perceive themselves to be at risk of HIV/AIDS and STD infections than those who were sexually inexperienced. While these responses reflect encouragingly accurate assessments of risk prevention, there was a high number of young people who gave inappropriate responses, such as 'I keep away from people who I think might have an STD/HIV' and 'I trust my partner'.

Explaining perceptions of risk

In some instances, young people's assessment of risk is appropriate in terms of their own sexual practices. However, it seems that young people's risk perception is intimately linked with specific personal beliefs. In testing Weinstein's 'unrealistic optimism' model of risk perception, Moore and Rosenthal (1991b) found a number of beliefs that predicted low perceptions of HIV/AIDS risk. These were: having a strong stereotype of a person living with HIV/AIDS; having a sense of personal control of whether they contracted HIV/AIDS; and believing, more than their peers, that the prospect of having HIV/AIDS was undesirable. In part, what appears to be happening here is that young people have linked HIV/AIDS to risk *groups* rather than risk *behaviours*. A strong stereotype of a person with HIV/AIDS is likely to be maintained because few young people have ever known or met such a person. Given that social representations of people with HIV/AIDS focus on gay men, injecting drugs users, and sex workers, and in the absence of personal knowledge of someone with AIDS, it is likely that the stereotype that young people hold will be of someone unlike themselves. This stereotype serves a distancing function, especially since it enables individuals to focus on differences rather than possible similarities (e.g. sexual practices) between themselves and those who are infected.

The belief that becoming infected is something over which one has control serves to reduce perceptions of risk and suggests that issues of mastery and the ability to take responsibility for one's own sexuality are important in enabling young people to assess their risk realistically. Finally, a sense of invulnerability may be fostered by engaging in risky acts that do not have immediate negative consequences. With the long lead time from infection to serious illness, this is especially problematic in the case of HIV infection. It is also true, given the epidemiology of HIV, that for most young people perceptions of low levels of risk are in fact accurate. This is not so for other STDs, as we have seen earlier. Moreover, for most other STDs, symptoms appear quite soon after the sexual encounter that leads to infection. While there are few studies that explore predictors of STD risk, in one (Moore and Rosenthal 1992a), higher perceived risk of STDs was shown to be associated with viewing this group of diseases less seriously and with the belief that one has little control over whether they are contracted. Stereotypes of a person with an STD did not predict perceived risk. The authors speculate that, unlike HIV/AIDS, it is more likely that young people know or know about individuals infected with an STD, which serves to reduce stereotyping of such people.

This last study is of interest because it sets HIV and STD risk perceptions in the context of other health-related risks (car accidents and cancer). In all cases, young people underestimated their risk relative to their peers but, importantly, the authors concluded that there was no evidence for unthinking 'invulnerability' on the part of their respondents. Rather, these young people made discriminating judgements that appeared to have a basis in reality about the relative likelihood of various events occurring. Further, although HIV and other STDs are sexually transmitted, young people rated the likelihood of their occurrence quite differently (and realistically), suggesting that the sexual nature of these diseases was not necessarily a block to evaluation of vulnerability.

The research to date, with the exception of this study, has examined perceptions of HIV and STD risk independently of young people's more general risk environment. There is evidence that sexual risk taking correlates with other risk-laden activities such as drinking, delinquent acts, and drug use (Jessor and Jessor 1977), but there is still the question of whether perceptions of risk associated with sexual activity form part of a more pervasive 'perception of risk environment'. In a recent study, Smith *et al.* (1995), unprotected sexual intercourse was rated as a high risk activity, along with driving a car while under the influence of drugs or alcohol, using inhalants, and taking amphetamines. Second-order factors suggested three over-arching and independent components to young people's risk perception: the perceived danger of a particular activity, the risk pay-off (which represents a balance between the pleasure or benefit obtained by engaging in the activity and the peer approval or disapproval that accrues from the activities), and the locus of control. By mapping the structure of young people's perceived risk environment, this study may provide a useful starting point for interventions to reduce adverse outcomes. If perceptions of risk in the sexual domain are embedded in a more generally structured risk environment, a broader-based approach to risk reduction may be an effective strategy. Certainly, recognition of risk is a positive step towards eventual change. The difficulty is to challenge the misguided beliefs that are associated with risky behaviours.

Young people consistently regard STDs, including HIV, as un-common occurrences. In this context, it is easy to see how young people arrive at the conclusion that they are not susceptible. The message that needs to be reinforced is that, even if the overall incidence of a particular disease is low, the behaviour of these young people renders them potentially vulnerable. Research has shown that most young people have not personalised the risk of HIV/AIDS infection, seeing the illness as a threat to others, not themselves. Moreover, in spite of high levels of concern about the presence of HIV in the community, concerns about HIV infection rarely figure in young people's decision making about safe sexual practices.

ATTITUDES: GOOD, BAD, OR INDIFFERENT?

Attitudes to STDs

While it is likely that attitudes to any disease will be negative, extreme attitudes of this sort may distort an individual's ability to think about a particular disease in a realistic way. As we have seen in Chapter 1, STDs have long been regarded as particularly unpleasant medical conditions, and ones that have been shrouded in shame and secrecy, presumably because of the assumption that they are associated with unclean sex. It might be hoped that in this day and age, with greater openness about matters sexual, these negative attitudes would have disappeared, or at least diminished. Not so. In a recent study of university students (Moore and Rosenthal 1995b), attitudes to STDs were more negative than to other, non-sexual medical conditions. In response to the question 'How would you feel if you got ...' (each of ten diseases), 'ashamed', 'unclean', and 'degraded' were the adjectives most strongly associated with the five listed STDs, including HIV/AIDS, while 'angry', 'depressed', and 'frightened' were the key descriptors of feelings about having other diseases.

So, in the liberated 1990s, STDs are still viewed as shameful and degrading diseases, unlike non-sexually transmitted diseases. Even if their symptoms are unpleasant or unattractive, we attach sympathy rather than censure to people who are unfortunate to contract diseases that are not transmitted sexually. It is interesting that the social construction placed on STDs is that they are somehow immoral, in spite of the value placed by our society on sexual attraction and, to some extent (at least for young men), sexual activity. The concern is that the negative social construction of STDs may impede the effectiveness or even the implementation of appropriate preventive education campaigns.

Attitudes to condoms

These campaigns have focused on the use of condoms as a preventive strategy. There is evidence that the message 'safe sex equals condom use' has been well learned (Lenehan *et al.* 1992; Stancombe 1994). In one study, safer sex was equated with condoms by 84 per cent of Scottish 18-year-olds, and with abstaining from specific sexual activities by only 2 per cent. Safe sex appears to be synonymous with condoms, although Stancombe reports that some worrying alternative meanings of safe sex are offered, such as having a 'clean partner', or 'no fun, boring sex life', and that few respondents equate safe sex with non-penetrative sex.

In the past, condoms have not been viewed in a positive light. In the pre-AIDS era, the pill was the preferred method of contraception, with condoms rating poorly in popularity (Chapman and Hodgson 1988; Morrison 1985). Reasons for negative attitudes to condoms vary. For some young people the issue is knowing how and where to buy the condoms, and feeling comfortable purchasing condoms, a particular problem for some girls (Bowler *et al.* 1992). Hence there have been suggestions that condom use may be increased by making condoms more available through, for example, the installation of condom vending machines (Kashima *et al.* 1992). For other young people the issue may not be the availability of condoms, but rather having the negotiating skills required to convince sexual partners to agree to using them. Insisting that a partner use a condom, or to insist on using it oneself, may be seen to imply that the partner has an STD. Rather than adopting the view that precautions are a sensible and necessary adjunct to sexual relations, the insistence on using condoms may be misconstrued as a lack of trust in the partner. This lack of trust may be difficult to reconcile with the idealised notion of sex that some young people, especially girls, cling to as occurring only between two people in a loving and trusting relationship (Buzwell *et al.* 1992).

Some young people dislike using condoms because they interfere with sexual pleasure and do not feel natural (Geringer *et al.* 1993; St Lawrence 1993). Yet others feel that carrying condoms 'just in case', will reflect poorly on their reputation. In particular, women may fear being labelled as 'easy' or 'a slut' if they carry condoms (Abbott 1987). It seems that there are a myriad reasons for unfavourable attitudes to condoms that are tied to the way in which young people view their sexuality.

One method of encouraging young people to discuss safe-sex issues and negotiate condom use is to normalise the use of condoms among sexually active people. There has been a push in Australia to reduce resistance to condoms with widely disseminated slogans like 'If it's not on, it's not on'. Unfortunately, we do not know if campaigns to promote a positive image for the condom have achieved their goal, although there is some evidence that attitudes have improved over time, especially among girls (Crawford *et al.* 1994; Rosenthal *et al.* 1996b). While a number of young people still have negative attitudes to condom use (Gallois *et al.* 1992a), encouraging reports from a number of Australian studies indicate that adolescents have a positive attitude towards using condoms and believe in the effectiveness of the condom as a precautionary device (Crawford *et al.* 1990; Moore and Rosenthal 1991c). Similarly, international reports present mixed conclusions about young people's attitudes to condoms. Some report that condoms are still disliked by many adolescents (Holland *et al.* 1990a; Worth 1989), while others claim that resistance to condoms is breaking down and that the necessity of condom use is being recognised (Abrams *et al.* 1990; Kegeles *et al.* 1988; Klitsch 1990).

Intentions and condom use

Even if attitudes towards condoms are becoming more positive, this will not necessarily result in increased actual or intended use. The links between attitudes towards condoms and intentions to use them are unclear (Boldero *et al.* 1992; Kashima *et al.* 1992; Moore and Barling 1991). Intentions to use condoms in the future have been associated with both positive and negative attitudes, yet actual (non-) use has been found to depend on young people's negative attitudes to condoms, that is, the disadvantages of using them (Boldero *et al.* 1992). In these studies, recognising the benefits of using condoms did not contribute significantly to actual condom use. This supports a report by DiClemente (1993a) showing that negative attitudes towards condoms, or the perceived costs associated with their use, were highly predictive of infrequent condom use. A more complex conclusion was reported by Dutch researchers who found that attitudes to condom use predicted actual use in a group of mono-gamous adolescents but not in a group who had multiple partners (Richard and van der Pligt 1991). It seems that the young people who were in monogamous relationships and who have negative attitudes to condoms deemed this AIDS precaution unnecessary, an option not available to those with multiple partners. It is of interest that, in the study by Boldero and her colleagues, attitudes to condoms *as AIDS protection* did not predict condom use. In other words, whether or not participants believed that condoms would protect them from AIDS had no impact on their actual condom use.

Attitudes to condoms: one dimension or more?

The relationship between young people's attitudes to condom use and sexual behaviour is not straightforward. Indeed, it may not be accurate or useful to polarise attitudes simply as either positive or negative. Clearly, attitudes to HIV/AIDS precautions are multi-dimensional rather than falling on one positive–negative continuum. In one study (Moore and Rosenthal 1991b), four independent dimensions were isolated: having negative attitudes to precautions, denial of risk of infection, the belief that one's partner has the responsibility for protection, and a fatalistic attitude to infection. These dimensions were related to gender and sexual risk taking in complex ways. Young men were more likely than young women to believe that responsibility for precautions belonged to their partner. Fatalism, the belief that personal behaviour is unlikely to influence outcomes, was found to be equally present in both sexes, however only for young men were fatalistic attitudes towards AIDS precau-tions linked to risky sexual behaviour. The important point to note is that people can have different patterns of attitudes on these dimensions and that there is a complex relationship between attitudes to AIDS precautions and risky sexual behaviour.

In another study (Robinson 1993), four factors emerged as underlying responses to questions about attitudes to condoms. These were: difficulty in negotiating condom use, implications of lack of trust, satisfaction with non-penetrative sex, and dislike of condoms. Among their sample of young women under 22 years of age, more than half reported having no difficulty in negotiating condom use with a partner. Similarly, more than half believed that raising the use of condoms with a partner did not imply a lack of honesty or trust. Finally, half of the under-18 group and three-quarters of the 18- to 21-year-olds reported some or a great deal of dislike for condoms. In summary, Robinson reports that the attitudes of young women (especially those under 18) are significantly more open to condom use and sex without penetration than their older peers.

Condoms and contraception

There is evidence of an overall decline up to the late 1970s in the reliance on male contraceptive methods and an increase in the use of oral contraceptives (Morrison 1985). In spite of the advent of HIV/ AIDS in the 1980s, most young people use condoms as a contraceptive rather than as an STD precaution (Donald *et al.* 1994; Robinson 1993; Traen *et al.* 1992). In one nationally representative American study of young men (20 to 29 years), of those who reported using a condom in the previous four weeks, half of the white respondents had done so only for birth control while a mere 7 per cent had done so for protection against HIV and other STDs. Oral contraceptives appear to be the contraceptive of choice for most young people, with condoms second (Chilman 1980; Tanfer *et al.* 1991). Thus, when young women are using other contraceptive measures such as the pill or diaphragms, condoms are unlikely to be used as an additional disease prevention measure.

FROM KNOWLEDGE AND ATTITUDES TO BEHAVIOUR

The gap between knowledge and behaviours, and the evidence that positive attitudes do not necessarily lead to safer sexual practices, have led researchers to recognise the complexities surrounding a sexual encounter. This is dealt with more fully in Chapters 4 and 5 when we consider the ways in which sexuality is socially constructed and the sexual practices that ensue. At the very least, however, it is now apparent that young people's unsafe sexual behaviour does not stem from a lack of knowledge about HIV/AIDS. For the most part, young people display high levels of knowledge about HIV/AIDS and while research has revealed some general gaps in young people's knowledge and slightly lower levels of knowledge among certain groups such as homeless youths, school dropouts, and some ethnic groups, it is clear that behaviour is not solely determined by knowledge. In contrast, young people's knowledge about STDs other than HIV is alarmingly deficient, confirming that much more effort has been directed towards educating young people about HIV to the exclusion of other STDs.

Condoms are seen as a critical element of the safe-sex message, but promoting condom use has proved to be a challenge. While there is evidence that some negative attitudes still persist, young people today, on the whole, hold more positive attitudes to condoms than did their peers in previous decades. However, positive attitudes do not necessarily result in increased intended or actual use. Condom use is not simply determined by whether young people are aware of their utility in preventing infection. Rather, there are many psycho-social and physical reasons for their not using condoms. By elucidating these factors, educational strategies can be more appropriately focused. For example, teaching young people how to become confident in their ability to deal with the practical aspects of condom use may be a necessary precursor to their adopting consistent condom-using behaviour.

As we have seen in Chapter 2, a substantial number of young people continue to place themselves at risk through their unsafe sexual behaviour, in spite of knowledge of safe-sex practices and modes of transmission of HIV. Research indicates that this is primarily because most young people have not personalised the risk of HIV/AIDS infection. Young people consistently perceive STDs, including HIV, as uncommon occurrences. They also believe that these negative, harmful events occur only to other people, especially to people who belong to highly publicised and stereotypic risk groups such as homosexuals, prostitutes and injecting drug users. These stereotypes of people with HIV/AIDS need to be broken down, with attention being redirected to the behaviours that place people at risk. While it may be true that HIV is not common among young heterosexuals at present, this is not so of other STDs. Targeting messages around the distressing possible long-term consequences of other STDs and the vulnerability of young people to these diseases may help to ensure greater uptake of safe sex.

4 Predicting sexual risk taking
Theoretical frameworks

EXTENT OF THE PROBLEM

Risk taking among adolescents and youth is a hot topic for researchers these days, not surprisingly given that young people's health is most severely jeopardised by their own risky behaviours. Irwin (1993) presents US data to show that the mortality rate increases by 214 per cent from early (10 to 14 years) to late (15 to 19 years) adolescence, with intentional and unintentional injuries from behaviours such as dangerous driving and suicide attempts accounting for this increase. In Australia, accidents rank equally with suicide as the major cause of death among the adolescent age group (Australian Doctor Weekly 1991). Millstein and Litt note that, 'In contrast to mortality among children and adults, adolescent mortality primarily arises not from disease but from preventable social, environmental, and behavioural factors. Behavioural factors also rank high among causes of morbidity in adolescents' (cited in Feldman and Elliott 1990: 433).

While it is not usual to think of death as an outcome of sexual risk, in the era of AIDS this is a clear possibility. Deaths from AIDS in the age groups 15 to 19 years and 20 to 29 years have been significant, and later death can result from youthful infection. Further, Grimes (1986) notes that females die in appreciable numbers in the United States and Australia due to the complications of STDs other than AIDS but that this fact receives little attention in comparison with the morbidity and expense issues associated with AIDS. Other serious and more common outcomes possible from sexual risk taking include unplanned pregnancy and the unpleasant symptomatology, curtailment of sexual life, or infertility that can be associated with STDs. Each of these outcomes may carry with it anxiety, guilt, social stigma, and unplanned and unwanted lifestyle changes.

SOME DEFINITIONAL ISSUES

The focus of this chapter is on sexual risk taking, but many writers stress the links between particular kinds of sexual activity in youth and other forms of unhealthy or maladaptive risk taking (e.g. Dryfoos 1990; Irwin 1993; Jessor and Jessor 1977). Metzler *et al.* (1992) found high correlations between unsafe sexual activity and smoking, alcohol and marijuana use in three independent samples of 14- to 18-year-olds. Moore and Rosenthal (1993b) showed links between sexual risk (multiple partnering, unprotected intercourse), smoking, and risky (fast) driving among older adolescents. It is important therefore to assess the role that general theories of risk taking play in helping to explain sexual risk.

A generally held belief about young people's risk taking is that it is deviant, leading to behaviours that jeopardise health and well-being. Teenagers engaging in these behaviours may be viewed as rebellious and alienated from the traditional institutions of society, especially the family and school. On the other hand, our society values certain forms of risk taking, as evidenced by the approval afforded to those who excel at dangerous sports, do brave deeds on impulse, make 'creative leaps' in science, arts or politics, are socially outgoing, or even daring in fashion. The issue arises as to where sexual experimentation fits in this scheme of things. One hallmark of adult adjustment is coping with sexuality and such skills do not arise fully formed like Venus from the waves. Experimentation with sexual ideologies and sexual behaviours therefore has an adaptive and life-affirming aspect of paving the way to the development of mature sexuality. The growth of both independence and the ability to form intimate relationships are also likely to be assisted by certain varieties of sexual experimentation. So, to what extent is youthful sexual behaviour to be considered a set of negative, 'at-risk' behaviours, and to what extent does it involve positive, adaptive risk?

To some extent we shall skirt around the answer to this question by considering, in this chapter, only unprotected intercourse as risky sexual behaviour. This is the behaviour most associated with unwanted pregnancy, and the transmission of AIDS and other STDs. Sexual behaviours that *may* pose psychological risks to self or others, such as early sexual debut, sexual exploitation (as victim or perpetrator), multiple partnering, 'deviant' sex and the like will only be considered to the extent that they correlate with unprotected intercourse. The question regarding the nature of what is healthy sexual experimentation thus remains unanswered, but we have defined one dimension of unhealthy experimentation. In the following sections, several theoretical models will be applied to the prediction of risk taking, and their success in the forecast of sexual risk taking, operationalised as unprotected intercourse, will be discussed.

The following quotations illustrate some of the elements of adolescent sexual risk taking, both subtle and not so subtle. Adolescents indicate through these quotations some of their beliefs about unprotected sex and their, at times, irrational or not particularly safe mechanisms for dealing with sexual risk. To what extent do the models described below deal with these issues and beliefs? We shall revisit the quotations at the end of this chapter as a form of evaluation.

1 *Do you consider the risk of AIDS?*

Yes. Every time I stick a needle in my arm.... I don't share needles, and I wouldn't screw anyone without contraception, unless I knew they were clean. *(Homeless adolescent girl)*

2 *Do you do anything about [the risk of] AIDS?*

Well sometimes I forget, you know, which really pisses me off, and then I start to worry. I think probably now that I have been talking about it, I will think more about it in the future. *How will you do things differently?* Maybe I won't just sleep with anyone. *(Homeless adolescent girl)*

3 *Would you ever have sex without a condom?*

Once I was pretty drunk and the next day I thought it was a stupid thing to do because I didn't want to catch any disease. *(Anglo-Australian adolescent boy)*

4 *Would you ever have sex without a condom?*

I wouldn't like to but I probably would if it came down to it. If you were really sure about the girl and she was on the pill or something. *(Anglo-Australian adolescent boy)*

5 *What method of birth control do you use?*

I think the pill would be the best to use. I think the condom would take away from the sexual experience. *(Anglo-Australian adolescent boy)*

THE HEALTH BELIEF MODEL (HBM)

The Health Belief Model (Becker 1974; Rosenstock 1974) proposes that preventive health action, such as regular medical check-ups, taking prescribed medication, or, in the case of sexual behaviour, consistent use of condoms for penetrative sex, can be predicted by a series of measurable beliefs and attitudes. These are (a) beliefs that one is susceptible to the disease in question, (b) beliefs that the consequences of the disease are severe, and (c) a balancing of beliefs about the effectiveness of the advocated health measures (benefits of taking action) against the disadvantages of their implementation (barriers to action). Later versions of the HBM (Janz and Becker 1984) hypothesise that the combined levels of susceptibility and seriousness provide the energy or force to act, and the perception of benefits (minus barriers) provides a preferred path of action. However a stimulus, in the form of cues to action, is necessary to trigger the decision-making process. These cues can be internal (such as pain or anxiety) or external (such as doctors' warnings or mass media campaigns). In addition, a motivational factor, namely the salience of health and illness for the individual, is postulated such that an individual's positive health behaviours depend on the value placed by him or her on maintaining a state of health.

The HBM has been applied to some areas of adolescent risk taking, such as dieting and exercising behaviour (O'Connell *et al.* 1985) and sexual risk (Rosenthal *et al.* 1992). Most supportive research with HBM appears to have been conducted with adult or child samples rather than adolescents, and describes the prediction of compliance to particular health routines, for example, having regular dental check-ups (Weisenberg *et al.* 1980), or protective behaviours such as taking the contraceptive pill for pregnancy control (Jaccard and Davidson 1972). Fewer studies have examined the success of these models in explaining the avoidance of unhealthy or otherwise risky behaviours, such as smoking or binge drinking. Effect size, that is, the power of the model to predict accurately the behaviour in question, has not been reported in many of the studies reviewed (Adler *et al.* 1992).

Research demonstrates that the model's predictive value in the case of safe-sex behaviours is limited (Becker and Joseph 1988; Hingson *et al.* 1990). An Australian study (Rosenthal *et al.* 1992) illustrates these limitations. The study demonstrated equivocal results, with the model failing to predict sexual risk with either casual or regular partners for young men or sexual risk with regular partners for young women. Although the model predicted young women's sexual risk taking with casual partners, only 13 per cent of the variance was accounted for, and the one factor contributing to the significant regression equation was perceived susceptibility to HIV/ AIDS. The authors concluded that rational decision-making models do not capture the essence of adolescent sexual risk taking, and that these behaviours need to be contextualised before a clearer understanding of this process can emerge. While beliefs about the seriousness of a disease, individual susceptibility to that disease, and the costs and benefits of preventive behaviours may be important, they must be considered alongside the contribution of other factors such as social context.

THE THEORY OF REASONED ACTION (TRA)

Ajzen and Fishbein's (1980) *Theory of Reasoned Action* postulates relationships between engaging in a behaviour and attitudes towards it, knowledge of its likely outcomes, and intentions with respect to carrying out the behaviour in question. In this model, intention to perform a behaviour is the immediate antecedent of that behaviour. Intention is predicted by two factors, the individual's attitude to that behaviour and his or her 'subjective norms'. Attitudes are determined by beliefs (or knowledge – both correct and incorrect, explicit and implied) about the behaviour, and the perceived costs and benefits of engaging in it (outcome evaluations), while subjective norms are a function of beliefs that significant others (for example, family and/or friends) think that the behaviour in question is appropriate, together with the individual's motivation to comply with these perceived norms.

For the example of safe-sex behaviour, condom use for any given sexual act would be postulated as predicted by intention to use a condom for that sexual encounter. This intention would be predicted in part by beliefs about the efficacy and desirability of using condoms balanced by the perceived disadvantages of their use, such as messiness, social embarrassment, and the like. These beliefs would be mediated by beliefs about the desirability of the outcomes of condom use, that is, protection against HIV/AIDS, STDs and pregnancy. Through such beliefs, Ajzen and Fishbein argue, attitudes are formed, in this case attitudes to condoms. Another dimension of influence on intention would be adolescents' ideas about whether their parents, friends, sexual partner/s, and other significant individuals or groups thought that condom use was a good thing. These ideas, along with the individual's motivation to comply with the perceived values of significant others, form subjective norms about condoms.

Research using this model tends to indicate what we all know about New Year's resolutions – that intention is not always predictive of behaviour. For example, among a group of 112 disco-attending young singles, about one-half indicated that their intentions to use a condom in a sexual encounter may not be carried out if they were drunk or drug affected, or because of being carried away by the passion of the moment. Several also indicated that they would lose their resolve if they 'thought their partner was safe', 'no one insisted', or the partner did not want to use condoms (Rosenthal *et al.* 1996a).

The TRA has been extended to include other factors, such as the extent to which the behaviour in question is under an individual's control. The theory of planned behaviour (Ajzen and Madden 1986) and its predecessor have been used in several studies of safe-sex practice among adolescents, but again with less success than in studies of other health-related behaviours. For example, Boldero and her colleagues (1992) asked sexually active young people to state their intentions, as well as answer questions regarding attitudes and subjective norms with respect to condom use. The sample then returned a second questionnaire after their next sexual encounter, indicating (a) whether they had changed their intention, (b) whether they had in fact used a condom in the situation, and (c) aspects of the situation that may have interfered with their intentions, such as alcohol use, type of partner (regular or casual), and level of arousal. The correlation between initial and later intention was very low, indicating that intentions were not stable, and the timing of their measurement is crucial is assessing the efficacy of intention as a predictor of behaviour. Further, there was only limited support for a link between intentions (initial *and* later) and behaviour, and even less support for the importance of attitudes and subjective norms in determining both intentions and safe-sex practices. Contextual features (communication with a partner, level of sexual arousal, and condom availability) on the other hand were important pre-dictors of intentions to use condoms and actual condom use, but even inclusion of these situational factors did not fully explain non-condom use among those with intentions to have safe sex.

The authors concluded that, while the model may be useful in predicting behaviours over which individuals have personal control (such as use of the contraceptive pill, or undertaking regular breast self-examination or a dental regimen), and that are private and not initiated in the 'heat-of-the-moment' of a sexual encounter, this is not so for condom use. Deciding to use a condom usually requires both parties to agree at the time of a sexual encounter and thus cannot be wholly predetermined, and is certainly not private. As with the HBM, failure to take account adequately of both the situational and social context limits the utility of this decision-making model in explaining sexual risk.

Overall, the TRA works relatively well in predicting adult behaviours that are premeditated and rationally governed (Ajzen and Fishbein 1980; Ajzen and Madden 1986), but like the HBM it is less successful in explaining actions in which contextual and emotional factors have a major role. In these cases, intentions are often thwarted or discarded. Such situational factors may be more likely to sway adolescents than adults, because of their lack of experience in dealing with contingencies. It is also possible that adolescents actually define risk differently from adults because they are less able to recognise the persuasive power of situations.

THE AIDS RISK REDUCTION MODEL (ARRM)

The AIDS Risk Reduction Model is a framework for the prediction of health-risk behaviour that has, unlike the previous two models described, been put forward specifically to assist in the understanding of risk behaviour relevant to AIDS (Catania *et al.* 1990). Three distinct points in the process of changing or reducing sexual risk-taking behaviours are postulated. The first is for individuals to recognise that their current sexual behaviour carries a risk of HIV infection, the second to make a decision to alter high-risk behaviour, and the third to overcome barriers towards implementing that decision. These points do not necessarily follow in an ordered sequence, nor are they necessarily irreversible. For example, an adolescent could recognise his or her risk of AIDS with some partners but not with others, or could change behaviour because of pressure from a partner rather than recognition of personal risk.

At each point, variables are postulated to influence outcomes. For example, recognition of risk is predicted to be affected by knowledge of how HIV is transmitted, perceived susceptibility to AIDS, and social norms concerning what constitutes risky behaviour. These variables heavily overlap or are directly equivalent to some of those postulated by the HBM and the TRA. Commitment to a decision to alter high-risk behaviour is viewed as consequent on attitudes to high- and low-risk activities, that is, a cost–benefit analysis of the positive and negative outcomes of altering behaviour towards safer options. Perceived self-efficacy, too, is a necessary precondition for behaviour change. For example, adolescents must feel confident enough to purchase, carry and manipulate condoms during a sexual encounter before they will commit themselves to the decision to use them on a regular basis.

Finally, actual behaviour change, as opposed to change in intention, will be enhanced by the young person's sexual communication skills – his or her ability to discuss condom use with a partner, for example – and the social support available from friends, family and health professionals to reduce risk behaviour.

The ARRM was designed basically to predict adult sexual risk behaviour, and its application to an adolescent population is an empirical question. Research support is available for various elements of the model. Some of this has been described in relation to the previous theories discussed, and some, such as the self-efficacy research, will be described in the next section. The full ARRM model was tested with a small sample of sixty-three adolescents aged 16 to 20 years by Breakwell and Fife-Schaw (1994), and it accounted for 30 per cent of the variance of condom use. The authors note that the social representations of sex reflected in norms and values override intentions in the explanation of young peoples' prospective condom-use behaviour. Another consideration is that developmental issues relevant to adolescence may need to be included for the model to be highly successful in predicting the behaviour of young people.

PSYCHOSOCIAL FOUNDATIONS MODEL

Levitt *et al.* (1991) propose a model that they describe as delineating the psychosocial foundations of adolescent risk taking. Five broad factors are postulated as predictive of risk behaviour. These are:

(a) lack of knowledge or inadequate understanding of risk and its prevention;
(b) inadequate risk-management skills (such as the inability to break a habit, or say 'no' to peer pressure);
(c) biological predispositions and personality traits such as a high need for stimulation (sensation seeking);
(d) socio-cultural factors that encourage risk taking, such as attitudes of significant others and the pressures they exert, or the lack of good models of decision-making;

(e) a lack of awareness of the personal meaning of risk, such as is manifest in a sense of invulnerability or a fatalistic attitude towards preventable danger, resulting from a complex interplay of the previous factors.

Because of the comprehensive nature of this model and its specific applicability to a youthful population, we shall consider each of these potential predictor variables in some detail. First, do young people lack the knowledge and understanding of risk and its consequences? Certainly, numerous educational programmes and public health interventions have been designed to teach adolescents about the harmful effects of specific behaviours such as smoking, drinking, drug use and unprotected sexual intercourse, but not always with great success. This issue was discussed in detail in relation to unprotected intercourse in Chapter 3, but the findings will be briefly recapitulated here.

In early research on sexual risk, a key assumption was that unsafe sexual behaviour stemmed from a lack of knowledge about the transmission of HIV. So if young people knew the consequences of unsafe sexual behaviour then they would not engage in such behaviours. Although research in the mid-1980s suggested high levels of ignorance about HIV, by the late 1980s the majority of American youths questioned knew the major modes of HIV transmission, and most misconceptions had apparently disappeared. Similar findings were evident for Australian youth. Yet higher levels of knowledge were not systematically related to safer sexual practices. Nor was knowledge alone a reliable indicator of behaviour change.

Becker and Joseph (1988) propose a threshold effect of knowledge, whereby a certain amount of information is needed for behaviour change, but over and above this, other factors come into play. For example, those who are clear about the risks that accompany certain activities do not always have the skills to implement protective or avoidant behaviours. Adolescents may believe, for example, that they cannot give up smoking even if they try, or that it would be too embarrassing or difficult to refuse to engage in risky activities if there was strong peer pressure to do so. While some young people may be overconfident about their abilities to avoid risk, others recognise their inadequacies in this area. Levitt and colleagues (1991) call this factor 'risk-management strategies', but it has been conceptualised in a range of ways, for example, as self-efficacy (Bandura 1982) or assertiveness (Yesmont 1992). By way of illustration, Hadley's (1994) study of adolescent alcohol consumption showed that poor risk-management skills, such as difficulty in resisting peer pressure to drink or inability to make realistic judgements about the personal effects of alcohol, were strong predictors of binge drinking. In the sexual domain, a study by Rosenthal *et al.* (1991) showed that significant proportions of sexually active adolescents were not confident about their abilities (a) to refuse a sexual advance by a steady partner if condoms were not available (20 per cent), (b) to buy condoms (12 per cent), (c) to carry condoms around 'in case' (28 per cent), and (d) to discuss the use of condoms with a partner if other contraception was being used (17 per cent). Yesmont (1992) predicted that assertiveness would correlate with three types of sexual precautionary behaviours. These were caution about engaging in sexual intimacy, inquiry about a potential partner's STD risk history, and frequency of condom use. The predictions were confirmed with a sample of 253 undergraduate students. Education about risk needs therefore to be aimed not only at increasing knowledge and understanding of what constitutes unhealthy or dangerous behaviour, but also at improving the necessary skills to enable young people to avoid or 'say no' to this behaviour, and to engage in more health-promoting alternatives.

Levitt and his colleagues' third factor implicated in risky behaviour is biological predisposition and personality. These authors argue that some people by their very natures are more likely to take chances, do dangerous things, engage in risky behaviours. They mention the trait of 'sensation seeking', which according to Zuckerman (1979; 1983) has a biological basis involving neurotransmitters in the limbic region of the brain. This trait, defined as the 'need for varied, novel, and complex sensations and experiences and the willingness to take physical and social risks for the sake of such experience' (Zuckerman 1979: 10), has been correlated with at least one risky behaviour: substance abuse among adolescents (Andrucci *et al.* 1989; Teichman *et al.* 1989).

The association between personality and risk taking was investigated in a novel way by Levenson (1990). He selected samples of adventurous risk takers (rock climbers), antisocial risk takers (residents of a long-term drug treatment facility), and prosocial risk takers, or heroes (police or firefighters decorated for bravery). Discriminant analysis produced two functions that correctly classified 98 per cent of the sample. Drug-unit residents had high scores on an Antisocial function, characterised by emotionality, depression, psychopathy, substance abuse proclivity and lower scores on moral reasoning. Rock climbers had high scores on an Antistructural function, characterised by sensation seeking and moral reasoning. Neither discriminant function characterised the heroes, who interestingly enough scored low on thrill-seeking, suggesting their motives for taking risks were not based on this variable. The authors conclude that each group represents a different type of risk taking, with different underlying personality dynamics. They ask whether further research might best concentrate on developing a more comprehensive taxonomy of different types of risks, which vary systematically in their antecedents. Once again we must consider where sexual behaviour might fit, and perhaps the extent to which unsafe sex for any individual is antisocial, antistructural or better classified on some other risk dimension.

Exploring further the relationships between risk taking and socially valued personality dimensions, we investigated the trait of venturesomeness (the desire to try new, exciting activities such as deep-sea diving or bungie jumping) in relation to risk taking among 18- to 20-year-olds across four areas (Moore and Rosenthal 1993b). These were sexual risk (engaging in unprotected intercourse), smoking risk (current smoking behaviour), driver risk (dangerous driving), and passenger risk (accompanying a dangerous driver). Venturesomeness, a trait with positive, adaptive overtones, was significantly correlated with each of the four risky behaviours measured. Further support for the idea that risk taking can show both an adaptive and a maladaptive face comes from a study by Chassin *et al.* (1989). These researchers showed that adolescents who engaged in high levels of 'deviant' behaviour often exhibited such desirable characteristics as independence, assertion and creativity. Silbereisen and Noack (1988) argue that an important part of adolescent development is the struggle for independence and self definition, a struggle that can be aided in certain circumstances by the young person engaging in mild levels of risky or even deviant behaviour. Sexual experimentation fits the picture of a set of behaviours that may promote independence and other positive characteristics while incorporating many risk possibilities.

A fourth group of factors postulated by Levitt and his colleagues as potent influences on adolescent risk taking is sociocultural variables. If the social mores are supportive and encouraging of particular behaviours, then these behaviours are likely to be more common. For example, if it is seen as 'adult' to smoke and drink alcohol, then adolescents will experiment with smoking and drinking and embrace these activities as rites of passage to adulthood. The adult generation, particularly parents, indirectly provide models of acceptable or unacceptable sexuality to their children, through what is witnessed on a day-to-day basis of their intimate relationships, such as level of warmth and affection, respect, tenderness or violence, etc. Except in dysfunctional families, the direct expression of sexuality is not modelled, but many parents provide information on these aspects of sex through 'heart-to-heart' talks, provision of books and magazines, and acceptance and encouragement of the role of schools in sex education. These days there is no shortage of media models, and while these often come across as highly attractive to youth, they do not always present the image of sexual relationships that responsible adults would like to put across to their children.

Young people receive mixed direct messages about sex from adults, and they are also influenced by them in a range of subtle ways. Feldman and Brown (1993) investigated the possibility that parents affect their children's behaviour through the socialisation of coping strategies and personality traits. They found that learned restraint – incorporating the ability to delay gratification, inhibit aggression, exercise impulse control, be considerate of others, and act responsibly – was a mediating factor in sexual risk taking in that low-restraint boys at age 16 had more sexual partners than those high on this variable. Thus parental behaviour outside the sexual domain may be just as influential in shaping children's sexuality as direct sex education, possibly even more so.

The youth culture as well as the family present influential sexual norms to adolescents. Some of these norms may be highly supportive of experimentation and risk taking. Young people may feel they jeopardise popularity and being part of the group if they 'say no'. Media representations of youth culture may model or even glorify unhealthy behaviours, such as sunbathing or dieting to excess. In the sexual domain, exploitative sex is often depicted in teenage videos and music.

An individual's social context provides for the learning of attitudes and values in relation to risk. Some of these attitudes and values are conscious and readily expressed; others may be held at a subconscious level, and are not easily recognised by the individual as affecting behaviour. Attitudes are not necessarily consistent with one another, or with resultant behaviour. Among young people, we found inconsistencies in sexual attitudes that meant that their general beliefs that it is a good idea to engage in safe sex were not always enacted. Various justifications for unsafe sexual practices were presented, for example that it would be detrimental to the relationship to ask a regular sexual partner to use a condom, or that condoms were somehow not as important if you were in love, or that you could 'tell by looking' if a potential partner was infected (Buzwell *et al.* 1992).

Finally, the meaning each adolescent attaches to risk will determine his or her degree of risky behaviour. This meaning will in turn be affected by the factors delineated above – knowledge, skill, personality traits and social context. The personal meaning factor is in part captured by an assessment of adolescents' beliefs in their vulnerability to the potential consequences of risky action. Elkind (1967) used the term 'personal fable' to describe what he argues is the widespread perception among adolescents that they are special, unique and invulnerable to the risks associated with their reckless behaviours. We found that young people did in fact consistently underestimate their level of risk, in the sense that most believed themselves to be less at risk of car accidents, lung cancer, skin cancer or STDs than an average person of the same age (Moore and Rosenthal 1992a). So for many adolescents, the personal meaning of risk is, clearly, 'it won't happen to me'. Bringing home the reality of that risk is partly a function of increasing knowledge and partly a function of personalising the message.

Perceived invulnerability, however, is not the whole story. A study of perceived risk of AIDS showed that among young people who were engaging in unprotected intercourse, and thus vulnerable with respect to HIV, two groups emerged (Moore and Rosenthal 1991a). There were those who did not recognise their risk, as discussed above, but there was also a 'risk and be dammed' group. These young people – mostly males – acknowledged their risky behaviour as such but went ahead anyway. Their reasons, though not assessed in the study, can be postulated through examination of both the research literature and case material. For some, it seems to be a case of the belief that life without risk is no fun: 'one crowded hour of glorious life is worth an age without a name', or in more contemporary terms, 'live hard, die pretty'. A second reason behind consciously reckless behaviour may be that some adolescents want to change their behaviours but lack the skills or persistence to do so. In support of this we found that those who saw themselves as most at risk of either skin cancer or STDs were those who felt they had little personal control over whether they contracted either of these diseases. For this group, educational interventions that facilitate a sense of personal mastery and teach directly the skills needed for safe behaviours would be ideal. Finally, there may be an association for some between the 'risk and be dammed' mentality and depression and low self esteem. The belief that one 'is not worth looking after so why bother' may be a reason why some young people take risks with their health and well-being. For these youths, the need to increase social supports and provide the opportunities for self-enhancement through meaningful and achievable goals is paramount.

DEVELOPMENTAL ISSUES

The models described above do not explicitly consider the specific characteristics of adolescence and the particular issues associated with this phase of development. However, there is increasing evidence that such factors make a difference. For example, Udry and his colleagues conclude that sex hormones, especially testosterone and androgenic steroids, have an important role in the onset of sexual behaviour in males and females, and other risk behaviours in males (Udry 1985, 1988; Udry and Billy 1987). Further, Irwin (1993) presents data that show that early adolescents have different perceptions of risk from older adolescents – a possible developmental change. Older adolescents tend to view the same behaviours as less risky than do younger ones. This may be associated with their more accurate assessment of risk; on the other hand it could mirror the phenomenon demonstrated in Weinstein's (1984) studies of adults, in which unpleasant risks were systematically underestimated (unrealistic optimism). The tendency for developmental researchers to saddle adolescents with antisocial and irrational coping strategies and behaviours really needs to be viewed in the context of modal adult development – some of these behaviours and strategies may be less of a function of adolescence than a function of emerging adulthood!

Several models have been proposed that integrate adolescent developmental principles with risk factors for the emergence of risk-taking behaviours (Irwin and Millstein 1986; Irwin 1993; Jessor and Jessor 1977). While these models focus on risk taking generally, rather than specifically on health-related behaviours, they do take into account intra- and inter-individual processes and influences, as well as the social context and the interactive nature of these three systems. In their general risk-taking model, Irwin and Millstein posit that biological maturation (the timing of puberty) has an impact on psychosocial aspects of development, including self-perceptions (body image and self-esteem) and developmental needs (autonomy, peer affiliation, intimate relationships), on cognitive scope, on perceptions of the social environment (such as the relative influence of parents and peers), and on personal values (such as independence and achievement). These variables are hypothesised to predict adolescent risk-taking behaviour through the mediating effects of risk perception and peer-group characteristics.

The model developed by Irwin, Millstein and their colleagues allows for an examination of a wide range of biopsychosocial factors and their association with health-related risk behaviour. Their model was adopted in some Australian research (such as the early work of Rosenthal and Moore) because it recognises the complex nature of the mechanisms underlying risk behaviour and includes not only endogenous factors but also exogenous, environmental determinants of behaviour. Moreover, the model is a developmental one, dealing with risk in the context of other adolescent developmental tasks. In spite of its complexity, the model is limited for our purposes because it focuses on risk without placing sexual risk taking within the context of sexuality, broadly speaking. An understanding of young people's sexual risk taking must include consideration of the nature of sexuality (both heterosexuality and homosexuality), the social norms that underpin sexual practices, and the understandings of sex that ensue – in short, social constructions of sexuality – to be discussed in more detail in Chapter 5.

Writings from anthropology have informed the work of Tacey (1994) and others, for whom adolescent risk arises from a developmental need for initiation and 'rites of passage' to mark the emergence from childhood. Tacey notes that modern society is devoid of meaningful rituals and causes, so youth invents its own in the form of reckless activity. He suggests that at different ages we have necessary rites of passage to attend to, and unhealthy risk taking is not a concomitant of maladjustment among adolescents, but of our sick society, which does not allow for these rites to occur in a meaningful way. Research that explores the meanings that sexual behaviour holds for today's youth may help shed light on the extent to which 'sexual recklessness' is indeed substituted for more healthy mechanisms for the attainment of adult status. As yet this is an under-researched area.

PHENOMENOLOGICAL APPROACHES

It is interesting that, in all the above approaches, the decision as to what constitutes risky behaviour has been made by the researcher, despite the fact that the importance of 'personal meaning' (Levitt *et al.*

1991) and risk perception (Irwin 1993) have been stressed as key variables in models of risk prediction. But adult conceptions of risky activity may or may not correspond with those of young people. In an attempt to investigate this issue further among Australian adolescents, Moore and Gullone (1995) studied risk from the subjective viewpoints of adolescents, with the aim of assessing their perceptions of what constitutes risky behaviour and how risk behaviours and risk judgements relate. Participants were 570 school-based adolescents, aged 12 to 17 years. The young people named risky behaviours perceived as common to similarly aged peers, then rated their own level of participation in these behaviours. The perceived positive and negative outcomes of risk were also nominated, and rated in terms of their perceived likelihood of occurrence and relative desirability or undesirability.

The sample viewed risky behaviours as smoking, drinking alcohol, dangerous driving, taking drugs, criminal behaviour, sporting risks, antisocial behaviour, minor rebellion (staying out late, lying to parents), school-related risks (playing truant, being impudent to teachers), and sexual activity. While there was a strong overlap between social consensus and adolescent perceptions of risk, adolescents did nominate some risk behaviours that can be classified as age related, such as rebellion against school authorities and parents. Further, age differences emerged in perception of risk, with older students more likely to mention drug taking and various sexual behaviours as risky, while the younger age group were more likely to nominate smoking and school rebellion.

Negative outcomes of risk were categorised as death, disablement, punishment and various social consequences, some of which could be interpreted as age associated, such as peer-group rejection. Pay-offs included pleasure, material gain and avoidance of negative outcomes. This last positive consequence, presented as 'getting away with it' or 'not getting caught', was a popular choice as one of the positive outcomes of many different kinds of risk taking. It is consistent with the notion that adolescents use risky activity as a form of independence seeking, although further research is needed to chart the extent to which such a mechanism is a characteristic of adult risk taking as well. Interestingly, getting pregnant or having a baby were nominated as both positive and negative outcomes of unprotected sex, showing that we cannot assume that outcomes socially designated as negative are necessarily perceived to be so for all adolescents.

A further finding of the study was a consistent pattern of

correlations between risk participation and outcome judgement, with perceived pleasantness and likelihood of positive outcomes and unpleasantness of negative outcomes strongly related to behaviour. The likelihood of the negative consequences was not, however, related to risky activity. In other words, adolescents engage in risky behaviours if they think there is a reasonable chance of pleasant outcomes, even if they are not very clear about what those outcomes are, over and above generally feeling good, and getting away with it. In addition, adolescents are less likely to engage in risky behaviour if they recognise potentially negative outcomes, but the likelihood of those outcomes is not a clear influence. The implication is that common adult emphasis on the dangers of sex (see, for example, Darling and Hicks 1982; Moore and Rosenthal 1991b) may not be the most effective strategy for dealing with adolescent sexual risk taking. Rather, a positive valuing of the pleasures and advantages of condom use may be more effective.

In summary, this study indicates that risk engagement in adolescence can be predicted by a rational-decision-making model if we use adolescent definitions of what is risky. It does not, however, take the next step of analysing the social and sexual context in which these perceptions develop, an issue that we shall explore further in Chapter 5. As a prelude to this, we return to the young people's comments quoted earlier in this chapter (page 55) to evaluate the extent to which the theories explicated above deal with young people's own individual rationalisations and explanations for their sexual risk taking.

RETURNING TO THE WORDS OF THE YOUNG PEOPLE

Adolescent number 1, a homeless girl, lives a risky lifestyle but sees herself as protected from AIDS if she is careful not to share needles (correct), and if her sexual partners are clean (incorrect, whether 'clean' is interpreted as not an injecting drug user or has its usual meaning). All the models described above could incorporate this mistaken belief into their set of predictor variables, as an individual or shared 'beliefs' variable.

Adolescent number 2, also homeless, is worried about AIDS but careless ('sometimes I forget') and could be unrealistic in her intentions ('Maybe I won't just sleep with anyone'). She has not internalised a plan to enable her to make future sexual encounters safe. Possibly Levitt *et al.*'s variable, 'risk-management strategies', most effectively captures what this girl is lacking. Neither the Health

Belief Model nor the Theory of Reasoned Action deals readily with situations in which the individual is ill-equipped for rational decision making, as in the case of this adolescent.

The third quotation, from the adolescent boy who neglected to use a condom because he was drunk, highlights the importance of situational factors in risk taking. In this case the situational factors are personal, but they can also involve social or environmental pressures. Few theories can (or do) incorporate all situational possibilities, but good theorising in the risk-taking area needs to take account of the commonness of certain situations, like alcoholic overindulgence, in the lives of adolescents. Qualitative research may help uncover some of the less obvious of these.

Adolescent number 4 shares some of the misperceptions incorporated in the first quotation. He might have sex without a condom if his partner was on the pill and he was 'really sure about the girl', suggesting that judgements about who is infected can be made on some basis of which we are left unclear – perhaps 'by looking' or through trust, two common strategies that teenagers use in these situations (see Chapter 5). While, ostensibly, decision-making theories can incorporate incorrect beliefs and misperceptions as part of their predictor variables, capturing the possible misperceptions behind what it means to be 'sure' about someone might be difficult to do with knowledge and belief surveys. This young man may well know all the right answers to what is good and bad practice with respect to HIV/AIDS, but when it comes to choosing a non-infected partner, there could be an implied message in his quotation that he will 'just know'.

Finally, adolescent number 5 presents an attitude towards condoms (they 'take away from the sexual experience') that could presumably be readily measured by a self-report questionnaire, and that fits neatly into all the models presented.

So are the theories adequate to explain adolescent sexual risk? The simple answer is that each adds important dimensions to this endeavour, but none is able to capture the whole experience of sexual risk. Realistically, theories can only act as summarising tools; a perfect predictor would be so complicated that its usefulness in allowing us to shape and influence behaviour would be lost. But theories need to be refined and changed as social situations change. Adolescent social mores are in a constant state of flux – the misperceptions and irrational beliefs of yesterday no longer influence today's young people, but a new set of misperceptions and beliefs takes over. For example, a commonly held belief at the turn of the nineteenth century was that sex with a virgin could cure syphilis, a belief of some influence to romantic young girls (see Gunn and Guyomard 1990). Finding out the new mythologies and social norms and factoring them into our education of adolescents is important in reducing the negative elements of adolescent sexual risk taking.

5 Myths and stereotypes
Young people's decisions to have and not to have safe sex

Considerable energy has been devoted to educating young people to adopt safer sex practices. We have seen that these efforts have not had a high success rate. Why? Sobo notes that:

> Programs in which educators didactically present facts about AIDS and HIV transmission do not increase condom use unless they speak to culturally salient concerns. This is because cultural constructions of HIV transmission and, more importantly, cultural constructions of sexuality – and all that it involves – condition perceptions of risk and so affect what HIV/AIDS educators call 'risk-education behavior' in the client population.
>
> (Sobo 1993: 456)

Sobo calls for the contextualising of sexuality education to take account of the range of underlying assumptions and discourses that influence how various sub-groups within the population construe their sexual lives. To achieve such contextualisation, we need detailed accounts of these assumptions and discourses, and their roles in mediating the safe-sex message.

Research on psychosocial factors associated with condom use in the early years of the AIDS epidemic concentrated on describing the levels of use, and correlating broad factors, such as demographic variables, knowledge about AIDS, and attitudes towards both AIDS and condom use, with safe-sex practice. In the previous chapter we saw the refinement of such studies through placing them in the framework of psychological theories of decision making, risk taking, and choice. Through this approach, some predictors of unsafe behaviour have been detailed, but they do not tell the whole story. If we are to understand youths' responses to the AIDS epidemic we must take account not only of knowledge and attitudes but of the broader social context in which sexuality is constructed and decisions about sexual behaviour are made. Several lines of recent research have been directed at uncovering some of the more subtle aspects of the sexual worlds of those in their teens and twenties, aspects that mediate the relationships between knowledge, attitudes and safe-sex practice. These will be discussed as myths and stereotypes about sexual relationships, which seem to surface when young people talk about their sexuality and its consequences. This chapter could well have been given the title that Sobo used as the subtitle of her article – 'The psycho-social benefits of unsafe sex' – because what we are looking at are the beliefs that support and encourage unsafe behaviour.

LOVE CONQUERS ALL

Sexual relationships that go beyond an initial encounter frequently develop through stages in which trust, feelings of commitment, and 'love' increase. The relationship changes from casual or 'new' to regular and steady. Correspondingly, caution about infection decreases (Wight 1992). Holland *et al.* (1990a) note that within a steady relationship, commitment is often indicated by the female beginning to use the contraceptive pill and condom use being discontinued. These researchers concluded from their interviews with young women that developing trust includes assumptions of monogamy. Persisting with condom use can be interpreted as undermining this assumption, therefore calling into question trust, commitment and the strength of the love relationship. As we have seen in a previous chapter, suppositions of monogamy are particularly dubious among young people, and have different levels of importance for males and females.

Further, even early in relationships, or in relationships unlikely to develop beyond casual encounters, young women may be particularly prone to 'trusting to love' (Rosenthal and Moore 1993). To believe otherwise flies in the face of social conventions about what is respectable behaviour for females. In spite of arguments that the 'double standard' is dead and gone, our research shows that young women are still far more concerned about their reputation than young men, and fear the disapproval associated with casual sex. Because of this, young women are likely to interpret casual encounters as something more meaningful and long term, so are less likely to interpret these as risky. Many young Australian women believe they can control their vulnerability to HIV/AIDS (and presumably other

STDs) by limiting their sexual activity to regular partners (Abbott 1988; Rosenthal *et al.* 1990).

Sobo's (1993) qualitative research on poor black women in an urban area in the United States describes a 'monogamy narrative' underlying non-condom use, which is very similar to the 'trusting to love' rationale for non-use of condoms described above. In the monogamy narrative there is recognition that many men cheat on their partners, but the idealised heterosexual union is one of faithfulness and trust. Admitting one's partner could be unfaithful damages self-pride and social position. It also damages the emotional comfort and security the relationship brings because it moves it one step away from the fantasy of ideal. Being cheated on brings shame and emotional hurt. 'Disinclined to experience pain or lose status, women deny the possibility of adultery in their relationships. Condomlessness helps them to do this as it implies fidelity' (Sobo 1993: 471).

Unprotected intercourse was interpreted by one woman as 'more romantic...special'. Sobo reports the following quotations from women interviewed in her study: 'It makes me feel like the relationship is strong and healthy and trustworthy and faithful'; 'We feel closer to each other without condoms'; '[With unsafe sex there is] nothing in between you both physically and emotionally. You are the closest to him that you can be.'

Galligan and Terry (1993) indicated from their study of 18- to 29-year-old university students that non-use of condoms is determined to a large extent by emotional concerns that are not factored in ahead of time when formulating the intention to use or not to use a condom. Disquiet about destroying romance featured strongly among these emotional concerns. Those who never used condoms with new or casual partners were far more likely to believe that their use 'would make sex seem like a business contract rather than a spontaneous affectionate act', 'would partly destroy the sense of trust and intimacy in the relationship', and 'would destroy the magic of freely relating to another'. For regular partners, these concerns about romance were much more likely to relate to non-use of condoms for young women. Young men who actually used condoms in regular partnerships thought they 'were more likely to ruin the special atmosphere of a sexual encounter and make it seem matter-of-fact', and 'would partly destroy my feeling that my partner was of special significance to me'. The authors surmised that these young males who identified a loss of romance associated with condom use with regular partners would apply strong pressure for their partners to change to a less intrusive contraceptive method.

The close links between the ways both men and women think about love and sex may allow sex to be interpreted as safe through its relationship with love. In a study by Rosenthal *et al.* (1996d), interviews with young single heterosexual women and men revealed an all-pervasive construction of sex in terms of love and romance, with almost all respondents repeatedly constructing their experiences of sex through these categories, as shown in the following examples (our emphasis).

Females

INTERVIEWER Describe your ideal *sexual* partner.

DIANE I don't think good looks are that important, I think much more that feeling that you *love* someone, friendship, mateship that's important.

INTERVIEWER What is the relationship between romance and *sex*?

TONI Well for me the only relationship is that *it is love* and romance.

INTERVIEWER Why do you have *sex*?

INGRID Um because I want to show my affection to the person that I actually am in *love* with them.

Males

INTERVIEWER If I say the word *sex*, what does it mean to you . . . ?

PATRICK When two people make *love*.

INTERVIEWER What is your idea of perfect *sex*?

DANIEL To be in *love* with somebody and to have a nurturing and loving relationship.

INTERVIEWER What is the relationship between love and *sex*?

CURTIS Um well sex is just *part of love*, it's another expression.

This invocation of love with sex is quite surprising given that these replies came from people who were at night-clubs and singles bars. Respondents were, of their own volition, participating in organised activities that implicitly and to some extent explicitly promote casual, short-term social and sexual encounters, yet they clung to more conservative notions of love and romance when talking about their experience of sex. The representation of sex as love appears to be a symptom of the social pressures within heterosexuality to define sexuality in a particular way. Unfortunately, as discussed previously, 'trusting to love' provides a barrier to safe-sex practice. For example:

INTERVIEWER   In what situations would you have sex without a
condom?

BECKY If I knew the person a minimum of three months. As long as I
trusted and loved him.

KATRINA To contemplate having unprotected sex with someone I'd
have to contemplate either being in love with them in the future
or being in love with them now.

Altman (1992a) has described why the 'love and trust' issue is less
likely to work against safe-sex practice for gay men. He argues that
there is a far higher acceptance of multiple partnering among gay
men than among heterosexuals, and that 'fidelity' in the sense of love
and trust within homosexual relationships does not carry the same
expectation that these relationships will be sexually exclusive. This
makes it easier to develop safe-sex practices, as couples can admit to
themselves that there may be risk of infection from other partners
without jeopardising their central relationship. Discussions about
how disease may be avoided are possible within this context. The idea
of 'negotiated safety' does not work in the same way for heterosexuals, for whom the negotiation tends to be around pregnancy
protection. Once this is ensured, the couple may believe there is no
socially acceptable avenue left for them to discuss disease protection
without calling the nature of the relationship into question.

BOYS CAN'T HELP THEMSELVES

Traditional gender-role expectations and mythologies are still prevalent among young people. The idea that male sexuality is an
uncontrollable and dominant force is seen by many young people as
the natural order of things. In our work we have found that young
people of both sexes readily endorse the conventional view that
males' but not females' sex drive is largely uncontrollable (Moore and
Rosenthal 1993a). Many teenagers believe that girls have greater
control over their sex urges because they are more responsible, or
because their urges are weaker than those of boys in the first place.
Some examples follow, the first from a teenage boy, the second from a
similarly aged girl.

1 *Can boys control their sexual urges?*

No, if you don't get a girl you go home and have a good old wank.
That's why we hate cockteasers so much.

It is often said that men are controlled by their dicks – is this true?

Bloody oath mate, it can make you do irrational things.

What are women ruled by?

Silly, stupid, romantic notions.

2 *Can boys control their sexual urges?*

Not really, no. They can be controlled by the girl, but they certainly wouldn't stop if they wanted something. Or they might if they cared about the girl and everything.

Can women control their sexual urges?

Yes.

It is often said that men are ruled by their dicks – is this true?

Some are – that is all they think about. Even though they might have morals against it, because they want it so bad they will just go for it.

What flows from this? Young men are let off the hook of responsibility because they 'can't help themselves'. Young women are expected to take an active and difficult controlling role, which is counter to the accepted norms of 'womanly' behaviour. For many young women, the ability to be assertive in a sexual scenario may not be easy or even possible. It may be in this context that unprotected sex occurs.

Additional weight is given to the sexual imperative for young men in a study reported by Goggin (1989). Goggin found that 18-year-old young men were more likely than their female peers to report high levels of sexual arousal and desire for sexual exploration. Conversely, young women reported stronger belief in sexual commitment than did young men. As might be expected, high levels of arousal and exploration were associated with greater sexual risk taking while high levels of commitment correlated with fewer sexual risks.

A variant of the 'boys can't help themselves' theme comes from Sobo's (1993) study of poor urban Afro-American women. She isolated from focus group interviews a 'wisdom narrative'. This narrative or discourse assumed that men's basic nature was to philander, to take sex when it was available, and not to worry about faithfulness. The wisdom aspect involved the women's ability to spot the con men and sweet talkers, and to choose a man who doesn't 'mess around' with other women. Such a skill was a sign of prestige in the community. In terms of protection against sexual disease, the implications of this narrative were similar to those of the 'monogamy narrative' discussed earlier. Demonstration of a woman's ability to choose a 'good' man was to indicate that condoms are not necessary – to use them suggests the inability to choose (and keep) the right man. Wight (1992) argues that this kind of gender stereotyping is particularly influential in whether condoms are to be used in the first sexual encounter. Men are presumed to be more experienced (Kent *et al.* 1990), or at least both parties feel they must act as if this is the case, because social norms do not favour young women advertising their sexual experience. To complicate matters, women have the role of deciding how far things will go, the assumption being that the male role is to wear down the woman until she agrees to sex (Holland *et al.* 1990b). While in the 1960s, most young women felt that 'birth control is a man's business' (Schofield 1965: 107), the widespread availability of the contraceptive pill changed the perception of responsibility so that females are now often seen as the ones to take charge of contraception. This can of course be done quietly and discreetly with the pill – young women's reputations are not compromised by something they can do in private, without prior discussion with a sex partner. Condom use is, however, not a private act and involves partners communicating and, tacitly at least, agreeing about their use. So young women may find themselves in a double bind of social norms – expected to take responsibility but not expected to advertise that they are ready for sex and experienced enough to be worried about disease protection. Catchy slogans aimed at encouraging women to take the initiative in safe sex ('Tell him if it's not on, it's not on'), miss their mark because they do not address this bind.

Some hard evidence for this comes from the Galligan and Terry study discussed previously. Fear of perceived negative implications of condoms was related to unsafe sex practice in this study. Those young people who never discussed using condoms were more likely to 'be afraid of being viewed negatively themselves if they had condoms available at the beginning of a sexual relationship'. They also thought that having condoms available carried negative implications for both men and women because it 'implied that they had had other sexual relationships', and that it 'might look like they planned to have sex beforehand'.

The traditional interpretation of masculinity offers men greater power than women in gender relationships. In the sexual domain this position is manifested by a masculine preference for controlling the initiative (Kippax *et al.* 1994). In an earlier study, Waldby *et al.* (1990)

found that young men disliked women who attempted to exercise control over when a sexual encounter occurred. These young men considered themselves to be the knowledgeable partner in a sexual encounter and were offended when young women tried to intervene. As Kippax and her colleagues point out, while this stance does not necessarily preclude safe sex, it does make it difficult for young women to have their say and be heard.

Pleck *et al.* (1993) showed that adolescent men who held traditional attitudes to masculinity indicated having more sexual partners in the past year, a less intimate relationship at last intercourse with the current partner, less consistent condom use, more negative attitudes to condoms, and a greater belief that it is a male responsibility to look after contraception. The valorisation of the masculine sex role in our society brings with it beliefs about the vital importance of male pleasure and the primacy of penetration in sexual relationships. Young women are as likely to buy into these beliefs as young men, and reject approaches to safe sex that they perceive as limiting to masculine pleasure, or uncomfortable with respect to the power status quo. Gender-role expectations and beliefs about reputation for both young men and women can act as influential barriers to safe-sex practice.

Consider the following responses from young single women aged 20 to 24, when asked if they had ever had sex when they did not wish to, and how it felt.

> Um, yes, yes. Pretty low, like I felt uncomfortable, even though I loved the guy it was uncomfortable to say, you know, you don't want to do it. Because I felt like, at the time, I was in a relationship with him – I felt, not obligated to, but if he wanted to, I felt maybe I should want to as well, you know?

> Oh, you just feel – not in a sense of being, like, forced sex – probably in a nice way – um, but I feel let down. Because, I mean, I know it's pretty obvious, but you know, if I'm tired or whatever, or I don't feel like it today... I feel let down that this person would still want it. I suppose I am pretty pathetic but I'm not in control of the situation enough to feel that I can say anything.

So these young women would prefer not to have sex in the situations they describe but, for a range of reasons, feel powerless to assert their needs. The implications for safe sex are not promising. But it is worth noting that this sense of powerlessness can affect young men as well, although they describe it differently. When women are sexually assertive, the pressure many young men feel to always be ready and eager for sex can make it difficult for them, too, to say 'no'. The following quotations are by young men aged 20 to 24, asked whether they had ever had sex when they did not want to.

> Yes. I can't really say how I felt. I was just there. I sort of did what was sort of expected. It's not like I felt imposed upon. I was just some place I'd rather not be at the time.

> Yeah. With bozo. Oh man, I was in bed, she comes up, starts playing, and I said – Look, just get on top. I just wanted to go to bed. She got on top. It was shocking. I hated it. I just hated it. I remember that night about a year ago – it was just shit. But now – a girl comes over the other day, she wanted to have sex. I said no. It was fucking weird.

YOU CAN TELL BY LOOKING

Among some young people, especially boys, we find a willingness to engage in unprotected sex with casual partners after making judgements about a partner's likely infection that appear to be based on the partner's appearance or reputation. Use of physical characteristics as a justification for unsafe sexual behaviour has been found in studies of young homosexuals as well as heterosexuals by Gold and his colleagues (see Gold 1993 for a review). To illustrate, some self-justifications used by young gay men in one study were as follows:

> This guy looks so healthy he can't possibly be infected.

> This guy seems so clean; he doesn't look at all grotty or dirty. So he can't possibly be infected.

> This guy's so beautiful he can't possibly be infected.

It seems that inferences about the likelihood of HIV infection (and possibly infection with other STDs) of one's partner, based on that partner's healthy, clean, and/or beautiful appearance, are not uncommon among young people. What might be the origins of such inferences? There are several possibilities. First, they may not know that, because HIV has a long incubation period, it is not possible to tell from appearances who is infected. Alternatively, they may be drawing incorrect inferences by generalising from frequently encountered diseases. Most diseases do, in fact, have short incubation periods, so it is often true that one *can* tell by looking. Both these possibilities are implausible, since few of these young people are ignorant of HIV's long incubation period (see Chapter 2). It may be that young people are simply drawing on the socially constructed equation of beauty with good health. Whatever the basis for this misconception, it is vital that adolescents and youth learn to look beneath the external packaging to the realities of HIV transmission.

A related idea is the myth that the people we know are too well brought up, too respectable, too clean or, ultimately, too like us to be at risk of infection. In one of our earlier studies of first-year university students, 33 per cent of the girls and 35 per cent of the boys agreed or strongly agreed with the statement 'None of my friends are the kinds of people who would be AIDS carriers, it's just not an issue for me' (Moore and Rosenthal 1991b). Stereotypes of people with AIDS or an STD conjure up, for many young people, images of prostitutes, promiscuous people, gay men, and other minority groups, and these stereotypes make the personalisation of risk more difficult to grasp, an idea discussed in more detail in the 'It can't happen to me' section later.

IT'S NOT SOMETHING YOU CAN TALK ABOUT

I don't want realism ... I'll tell you what I want. Magic!
(Blanche Dubois, in *A Streetcar Named Desire*, Williams 1957: 178)

so much is said by tone of voice or facial expression that words are often secondary.
(from a sex manual by Masters and Johnson 1970)

Condoms are such horrible things, and to put one on destroys the magic of sex. Here we are on cloud nine: how can we suddenly interrupt everything just to get a bit of rubber out and roll it on.
(from Gold *et al.* 1991: 273)

Wight points out that:

There is a gap between clinical-sounding sexual terminology and vulgar colloquialisms (Lee 1983; Spencer *et al.* 1988) perpetuated by the taboo against the explicit discussion of sexual behaviour in the media. It should not be surprising, then, to learn that in a sexual encounter there tends to be very little verbal communication during the transition from sexual intercourse being a possibility to it becoming a reality (Kent *et al.* 1990). In fact ambiguity is often deliberately maintained.
(Wight 1992: 12)

Much sexual communication is of course non-verbal, which leads to ambiguities in interpretation when the issue is one on which a decision must be made, such as whether to proceed with sex, change an activity, and/or introduce a condom. Couples often do not decide to have sex verbally, but through action. The introduction of a condom into the situation indicates an assumption that sex *will* occur, before penetration has been attempted. There can be no escaping, then, the need to decide consciously whether to have sex or not – the ambiguity, which may be perceived as heightening romance, passion and spontaneity, or reducing personal responsibility, is removed. The desire for such ambiguity and 'magic' may therefore mitigate against the 'clinical' discussion of disease protection.

Cline *et al.*'s (1992) study of college students showed that only about 6 per cent of their respondents talked to their partners about condom use, although two-thirds had discussed AIDS in a more general way. Most frequent reasons for not discussing AIDS or safe-sex practices were embarrassment, 'did not know partner well enough', 'ruin the mood', and 'things happening too fast'. These reasons, say the authors, focus on concern for preserving self-image and for preserving the imminent sexual encounter. The implications for condom use are that, when partner communication is low, condom use will be jeopardised. In fact, Boldero *et al.* (1992) found communication with a partner was a more important predictor of actual condom use among tertiary students than either attitudes to condoms or knowledge about HIV/AIDS.

Communication with a partner about sex has another important function. It allows for discussion of a partner's sexual history, so that informed decisions can be made about the need for protection. Qualitative research suggests that few young people discuss their sexual histories before first intercourse. 'Those who do discuss each other's sexual past do so for reasons to do with the relationship rather than through fear of infection, so that it is unsurprising that they learn little to inform them of their partner's HIV status' (Wight 1992: 13). Ingham *et al.* (1991) suggested that one reason for young women not asking partners about past sexual history had to do with being sure that their own sexual behaviour together would remain confidential. For a boyfriend to reveal his past would destroy that trust.

Among young gay men, Gold and his colleagues found self-justifications for non-condom use frequently centred on fears of making a negative impression on a partner. What seemed to be felt was that producing a condom would communicate all sorts of other things apart from the desire for safe sex. Examples given were that to use a condom might communicate to a partner that you were promiscuous, sexually boring, or a 'wimp', in the sense of not being 'man enough' to take a risk (Gold *et al.* 1991). These self-justifications again underline the multi-layered nature of sexual communication, in that each act can be given many meanings and interpretations, which, if not discussed in words, are readily misinterpreted.

I'M ON THE PILL

Wight says that all recent qualitative studies in Britain show that condoms are used primarily as contraceptives (Frankham and Stronach 1990; Holland *et al.* 1990a; Ingham *et al.* 1991; Kent *et al.* 1990; Scott and Griffin 1989). When young people move into more regular relationships, the girl is more likely to go on the pill. The contraceptive function of condoms is then superfluous, and their role in protection from infection is apparently dismissed as no longer necessary as well. Sobo's focus groups indicated that a man requested to use condoms might respond coercively: "'Baby, don't you take birth control?" If a woman does have another method of contraception that settles the issue. A cognitive shift takes place and the original prophylactic intent is forgotten' (Sobo 1993: 474).

An interview study of ten young heterosexual couples, by Gurien (1994) in California, suggested that couples may slide between an understanding of 'safe sex' as protection against AIDS and STDs to an understanding involving protection against pregnancy. This slide in meaning becomes a comfortable one as the couples settle into their relationship, and interpret disease protection as a non-issue for them. The following comments about the meaning of safe sex illustrate the kind of thinking that appears to be occurring:

I think we have safe sex because in the sense that I'm not pregnant, but beyond that I don't know.

We don't use condoms because I'm on the pill.

Gurien noted that although couples were not asked directly to talk about pregnancy, there was far more concern expressed about this topic than about disease. She states that 'Although no one ever mentioned a fear of contracting AIDS/HIV, the fear of an unwanted pregnancy was pervasive' (Gurien 1994: 13). For example:

We have both been very concerned about pregnancy. That's probably why we're very safe.

Everything's going fine except [she] forgets to take her pill now and then which is a really huge 'no no'.

The issue of trust is again important here. Young people who have made a commitment to a close, intimate relationship, and who have made sure of pregnancy protection through use of the contraceptive pill, may feel threatened by the implied message in continuing to use condoms. The message is that one or other partner has not 'come clean' about past relationships, or is currently being, or thinking about being, unfaithful. Interestingly, in Gurien's study, trust-related reasons for not practising safe sex were overwhelmingly provided by the men, who clearly prided themselves in being able to discriminate between high- and low-risk partners. Cline *et al.*'s (1992) study, discussed in Chapter 2, indicating that both men and women will lie about their past sexual behaviour to protect their relationships, makes the confidence of these young men appear misplaced.

IT CAN'T HAPPEN TO ME

Most adolescents have not personalised the risk of HIV/AIDS, or indeed any STDs, seeing these illnesses as a threat to others, not themselves. Much has been made of teenagers' perceived invulnerability to unpleasant events and their belief that, although others may suffer the consequences of dangerous and risky actions, they are somehow immune. It is certainly true that a significant number of young people we have questioned believe that they are not at risk of HIV or other STDs, even when their behaviour suggests otherwise (Moore and Rosenthal 1991a, 1992a). Of course, the illusion of invulnerability may be encouraged when risky acts have no immediate negative consequences. Adolescents who repeatedly engage in unsafe sex without becoming infected are, not surprisingly, likely to deny the riskiness of that behaviour.

Another factor is that many young people have a stereotyped view of people with AIDS. Young people may link HIV/AIDS and possibly other STDs to risk *groups*, rather than risk *behaviours*. It has been thought that the stereotype is likely to be maintained because relatively few young people know or have even met a person with AIDS. However a recent study suggests that adolescents who do know a person with AIDS will *not* have higher levels of worry regarding a personal vulnerability to HIV infection (Zimet *et al.* 1991). In the case of STDs, the shame associated with these conditions means that even if one has met individuals with these conditions, they are not likely to readily discuss or admit to this.

Naïve social constructions of AIDS involve ideas about the type of person who will become infected, including homosexuals, intravenous drug users, and prostitutes. If young heterosexuals have no personal knowledge of an infected person, they are more likely to hold stereotypes of someone unlike themselves. As we determined in Chapter 3, this stereotyping allows young people to feel different and distant from individuals they perceive to be at risk. Outcomes include ignoring the possibility that some or even many of those who are infected may not fit the stereotype, or concentrating on superficial differences between themselves and the stereotype, thus failing to see fundamental similarities (such as in sexual behaviour).

One example of the misuse of these stereotypes is the idea that 'safe sex is for gays'. Young heterosexuals may associate HIV with homosexuality, and, within that logic, condoms as protection against HIV are also associated with homosexuality, as illustrated by the quotation below from a 16-year-old male:

Will AIDS affect how you go about sex in the future?

Well, I don't plan on turning gay, so I don't think ... I mean it will probably become more and more, but I don't think I will be at high risk. But it is something to be aware of.

As well as the 'it can't happen to me' phenomenon, other types of magical or superstitious thinking associated with condom use have been isolated by Gold *et al.* (1991) in their study of gay men. They found a kind of mental bargaining sometimes used as a justification for unsafe practices, wherein the young person reasons that he has been 'good' in the past (or will be in the future), therefore deserves to be protected during the occasional slip-up. Items such as 'Most of the time I'm careful, but I can't be perfect – it's only human to break out occasionally', or 'I'll have one last fling and only do safe sex from then on ...' were examples of this sort of reasoning. Ideas about the fallibility of the medical profession and AIDS experts, and the belief that one had a particularly healthy immune system therefore would be resistant to HIV infection, were also justifications for not using condoms in this sample. These justifications rely on beliefs that one is special and not prone to the risks that beset others (who act similarly), and is another example of the phenomenon known in the adolescent literature as 'the personal fable'.

I DON'T CARE WHAT HAPPENS

Fatalism, too, represents a kind of risk denial. There is a rejection of responsibility for the consequences of one's action. So the worst might happen if I take risks with unsafe sex, but either 'that's life' (there's nothing I can do about it, I have no control over the matter), or 'it doesn't matter anyway' (I am worthless, so what happens to me is immaterial). In fact, 7 per cent of girls and 11 per cent of sexually active boys in our study of first-year college students agreed or strongly agreed with the statement, 'There's a chance I could get AIDS, but there's nothing I can do about it', and 6 per cent of girls and 14 per cent of boys similarly endorsed the sentiment, 'Life is full of risks and AIDS is just one of them; if you don't take any risks, you don't have any fun' (Moore and Rosenthal 1991b).

Sobo (1993) noted that some of the poor black women interviewed by her team talked about their beliefs of others' perceptions of their worthlessness. These perceptions were internalised and lived out in practice, through disregard of sexual disease protection. Another interesting point made by this researcher was that personal responsibility can be limited through conspiracy theories, leading to a fatalistic outlook. The belief was held by some of her sample that AIDS was a racist plot to eliminate Blacks (for example, by the CIA). Farmer (1992: 247) describes such conspiracy theories as a rhetorical defence employed by powerless victims. If such a plot is true, then the targets of the plot cannot be blamed for the outcomes of their behaviour, and any attempt to take control of matters against such powerful and devious forces is futile. Similarly, if the promotion of condoms is viewed as an adult 'plot' to discourage young people from having sex, the related messages about STDs and AIDS can be more readily rejected.

One of the features of poverty, homelessness, or any form of deprivation may be that the benefits of unsafe sex (pregnancy, closeness, pleasing another) are perceived as outweighing the disadvantages. '[T]he only way not to do worse . . . is to take risks to do better' (Wildavsky 1988: 226). This sort of fatalism may affect groups of young people who are disaffected by their status and prospects in life, predisposing them to risk-taking behaviour.

DANGEROUS SEX IS MORE EXCITING

Adelman (1992) argues that the term 'safe sex' can be construed as an oxymoron if, as some writers suggest, danger constitutes a major element of sexual excitement. If unprotected sex is perceived as risky – and this is how it is currently described – then the promotion of safe sex can be seen to mitigate against arousal, excitement and, ultimately, pleasure. One potential way of breaking this nexus between pleasure and danger, according to Adelman, would be the eroticisation of safe-sex talk. Currently the discourse surrounding such talk is highly moralistic (for example, 'Just say no'), and may be effective in changing *intentions* about sex, but ineffective in situations of high arousal.

Public and private discourse about sexuality stresses the discourse of desire, but sex educational programmes for teenagers appear to ignore it completely, according to Fine (1988). Young people feel the excitement of sex, and it is emphasised in media portrayals, but no one talks about safe sex and sexual excitement in the same breath. In fact, more common is the link between 'risking all for love' (danger) and thrilling, passionate sex (desire). The depiction of spontaneous sex and sex in unusual places are common themes in movies and novels, themes that turn up as part of our (condomless) fantasy life, as in the descriptions offered by these young men in a study by Rosenthal and Moore (1995).

Would you be able to describe your sexual fantasies?

Um, I like . . . I always fantasise about having sex in a public place, or at a place . . . not actually being viewed by people, but somewhere you might get caught . . . in a park, or a street maybe, in an alleyway, or something like that.

The only fantasy I've had is probably I want to make love in an aeroplane at 30,000 feet. But yeah . . . I suppose the idea of being surrounded by so many people and you sneak off somewhere in a quiet corner and um . . . just being in flight, I suppose, it just turns me on.

Um, I guess in the shower, and in the bath.

None of these fantasies could readily incorporate condom use. If safe sex is construed as boring, conservative, prosaic sex, its uptake will be particularly limited among young people who are still experimenting with sexual possibilities.

CONDOMS ARE UNRELIABLE, SO WHY USE THEM?

Although research shows that attitudes towards condoms seem relatively positive among young people, we have been struck by the number who comment on condom unreliability when we talk about safe sex to various groups. Everyone seems to have a horror story about someone they knew for whom the condom broke or fell off, with dire consequences. These stories, told as often by adults as young people, seem to have reached the status of urban myth. Unfortunately, the conclusions drawn can be along the lines suggested in the title of this section – condoms are unreliable so why use them at all.

What does research say about this matter? Under laboratory conditions, the condom has proven impermeable to HIV (Van de Perre *et al.* 1987). But user error or variations in product quality can lead to condom breakage or slippage. In a nation-wide Dutch study, de Graaf *et al.* (1992), assessed the failure rate of condoms over periods of six and twelve months with prostitutes and clients respectively. They showed the breakage rate to be a low 0.8 per cent for prostitutes and 1.5 per cent for clients, with failure rarely attributed to condom quality. Rough or prolonged intercourse, incorrect handling, or insufficient use of lubricant were the major causes cited. A condom slipping off before or after ejaculation was an even rarer event than breakage. Such low failure rates may increase among a youthful population because of their inexperience, but they are clearly no cause to abandon the condom and substitute no protection at all. The citing of condom failure as a reason for their non-use among the sexually active would seem an illogical and indefensible strategy in the light of these data. It is a strategy nevertheless not confined to young people. The Dutch researchers whose work is described above found that certain groups of *adult* clients of prostitutes used doubts about condoms' safety as a justification for their non-use, for example, 'Even with a condom you don't know for sure', or 'They often rip' (Vanwesenbeeck *et al.* 1993: 87).

CONCLUSIONS

So, condoms are unnecessary or downright insulting if you love and trust your partner. They interfere with romance and spontaneity. It's too embarrassing for a girl to insist on their use, because it could appear that she was promiscuous, and certainly unfeminine.

Sometimes boys slip up on good intentions to use condoms, but they can't help it, and anyway 'real men' can pick a clean girl with a good reputation and/or are not wimps who worry about infection. Even if couples think they ought to discuss condom use, it is too difficult to bring up the subject, it gets in the way of the relationship, and in interactions between the sexes it is important to keep some things to yourself, such as the occasional infidelity. Being on the pill means the girl won't get pregnant, and let's face it, that's the biggest worry. AIDS only happens to other people – not to normal, regular people like us, with normal regular friends and lovers. Life's short, why not enjoy it while you can – too much caution could make sex pretty boring, and, to cinch the argument, condoms often break or slip off, so why bother?

In a nutshell, those are the myths and stereotypic ways of thinking that we have summarised in this chapter. They support non-condom use in a pervasive and subtle way, often not even recognised by the young person, who may give all the 'right' answers on a multiple-choice questionnaire about attitudes to safe sex, yet still be an inconsistent condom user. Much of this material has been uncovered through qualitative research methodologies, such as in-depth interviews, and may not be readily discernible in studies using more direct approaches. Some of the constructions of sexuality and life in general that uphold these myths have found support from more traditional methods, such as the Galligan and Terry (1993) study indicating the moderating effects of beliefs about love, romance and reputation on condom use. The generality of others is still to be tested, although in a sense what matters is not how many use these rationalisations for non-condom use but that they are used at all.

6   A matter of policy

At a secondary school in rural Australia in 1992, there was a state-of-the-art sex education programme that resulted in students being well informed about the need for safe sex and interested in the notion of practising it, yet anecdotally teachers were aware that condom use was low. Further exploration led to the awareness that the major barrier for these young people, who appeared willing to practise safe sex, was the difficulty of maintaining some semblance of privacy when everyone in the town knew who had purchased condoms, how many and how often. They experienced this as exposure beyond the bounds of the acceptable. It turned out to be a matter easily remedied in that the school council, when briefed about the problem, readily agreed to a policy that allowed a discreet supply to be available at the school and dispensed in a way that ensured students' confidentiality.

Just before the system came into operation, in response to public debate from other quarters, the state government announced that it was now a matter of public policy that condoms would not be available in government schools. So the school was obliged to abandon the scheme that it had concluded was critical to protecting the sexual health of their young people and to explore other ways of dealing with the issue or to revert to the unsatisfactory situation they were in before (Ollis 1995). This story demonstrates the sense in which policy can create the capacity for public opinion to have significant impact on the lives of individual young people.

Policy is official writ about how a nation, state, community or institution has decided to proceed, for example, in relation to HIV/ AIDS and STDs. It determines how these diseases will be discussed, prevented and managed by whom, and for whom. Policy at any level within a democratic society is developed with the co-operation of the stakeholders (or those stakeholders who have the most power at any time) and involves a formulation of a position that gives voice, priority and legitimacy to the resolution of a series of usually conflicting needs.

Policy in the area of sexual health is developed in the nexus of the conflict between public health demands and the desire for the protection of innocence, privacy and silence about sexual matters, and as such evolves within the same debate as sex education for young people, usually indeed gathering all these educational issues in its net.

STDs have traditionally been managed and legislated for under a disease-focused model based on what is now referred to as the 'old public health'. This model concentrates on locating diseases within individuals, and it attempts to protect public health by naming, categorising and taking control of infected individuals, making arrangements for restricting their potential movement. Where possible such individuals will be treated and cured (as in the case of tuberculosis (TB) management) or at least will be subjected to surveillance, sanctions and punishments that attempt to ensure they do not pass on the disease. In the case of STDs such an approach fed into community preparedness to accept their domain as pertaining to 'otherness' and immorality, from which 'normal' people were entitled to protection. HIV/AIDS has provided a critical challenge to this approach. At the simplest level, society has been required by the spectre of a deadly and incurable disease that appeared somewhat more intransigent to moral exhortations and recriminations than were its successors, to look with an enhanced tolerance on homosexuality, drug use and extramarital intercourse, bringing them into the arena of public scrutiny and debate.

The evolution of the 'new public health' first became visible in public-health movements around the world in the latter half of the twentieth century, culminating in the United Nations adopting in 1981 World Health Organization (WHO) global strategies to ensure Health for All by the Year 2000 (WHO 1981), and the development of the Ottawa Charter for Health Promotion in 1986 (WHO 1986). The WHO definition of health was extended beyond the simple absence of disease, and the domain of health management and promotion moved beyond the treatment and management of illness to include a spectrum of issues pertaining more to social and economic well-being and the social context in which health-related behaviours take place. This movement coincided fortuitously with the growing awareness of the global pandemic of HIV infection, and set the scene in which policy developed to address the new disease could take account of a wider social context particularly appropriate for sexually transmissible disease.

Adolescents, however, are seldom part of the policy development process (Wells 1992). As the majority of them are without a vote, they must rely on the commitment of parents, teachers and other concerned advocates to represent their best interests at a national level. The vexed issue of 'best interests' itself is interlaced with multiple agendas that each of these advocates may wish to pursue. A church group, for example, may present, in line with its own policy, the 'best interests' of adolescents as being met by forms of protection from knowledge about or pressure to engage in sexual activity. A position paper on 'rights, duties and obligations' as they relate to sex education, prepared by the Baptist Church states that:

> It is quite clear that sex belongs within a permanent heterosexual relationship. Sexual relations outside this relationship are disobedient to God's intention. Such sexual practices are sinful – whether they are heterosexual, homosexual or bestial practices. They are included for condemnation with other issues of social injustice in Deuteronomy 27: 15–26.

(Carmichael 1995: 1)

Information would then be presented with this end in mind. A different agenda, perhaps from a youth service, may defend the right of young people to be given information and support in order to make decisions about sexual behaviour for themselves, without pushing them in one direction or another. Whichever line is taken, it remains clear that it will not be young people themselves, except in somewhat tokenistic ways, who will determine the ways in which policies impact on their sexual health. Instead they will be relying on the experience, judgement and moral stance of their seniors to help or hinder their sexual growth.

ELEMENTS OF GOOD POLICY

A policy, whatever its content, that has a chance of successfully addressing the issues involved in managing and preventing STDs will be one that has arisen out of a process of community development, and in which all stakeholders have a high degree of ownership. There is little point in putting energy into attempting to implement a policy decision that does not have the interest and support of those who are most affected by it. Top down, 'for their own good' decisions, which characterise the old public health, have a history of very limited success. Such policies often gave immense power to individuals in authority to curtail the activities of supposedly infected others for the good of society. A rather comic illustration of this exists in the old Victorian Health Act, which was in force as late as 1988, by which tram conductors were empowered to eject from trams anyone they suspected of having an infectious disease. Nevertheless, attempts to take such an approach, based on the restriction of infected individuals in the delicate area of sexual health, abound (the threatened closure of the San Francisco bath houses in 1983, for example, to stop gay men having so much sex). This directive, even punitive approach, which does not take account of needs and social meanings beyond the narrow disease-prevention imperative, is even less likely to be effective when it relates to the private area of sexual behaviour and when it comes to policies that seek to prescribe certain behaviours to young people.

It is difficult to know whether, in the case of young people, it is better to deal with sexual health as a separate and significant issue, or to include sexual health in a comprehensive health policy covering a spectrum of health issues. Few countries have policies on young people's health as well developed as the current policy of the US Congress (Congress of the United States, Office of Technological Assessment 1991). This policy offers a two-pronged approach to HIV/STD prevention, seeking to support and strengthen sources of information and service provision attractive to adolescents and to foster improved data collection and relevant research. The broad-based nature of this adolescent health policy places sexual health commendably in the context of adolescent development and the plethora of other health issues that arise as part of it. However, in its adherence to a fairly medical and service-based approach, it also constructs the means by which sexual health can be buried so that it is less contentiously absorbed into issues of appropriate service provision. This means there need be no explicit direction about how sexual health for young people must be handled, but that it can become one of the many issues that services are required to address with discretion and sensitivity. There remains a need to recognise that services have the same constraints imposed on them as does the wider society, and other policies and legal sanctions can determine their real capacity to carry out effective STD/AIDS prevention.

A CASE STUDY: AUSTRALIA'S NATIONAL HIV/AIDS POLICY

Many policies at a national level have a major impact on the lives of young people, or at least have the potential to do so, without necessarily naming them in a target population. The sexual health of young people barely rated a policy mention at any level until the advent of HIV/AIDS, which required a rethinking of strategic approaches across the board. Governments now had to deal with a disease for which behaviour change was the only possible control measure and so had to gain the co-operation of sexually active people, many of them young, and ensure that they were not alienated, rejected, criticised or disenfranchised for fear of the health consequences. Australia's two national HIV/AIDS strategies, which name sexually active young people as one of their target groups, are an interesting case to examine in order to discern those elements of policy most likely to be useful and effective in the sexual health area. This is because Australia had the opportunity to observe the experience of other countries where the disease became more rapidly established, and where the responses were more crisis driven, piecemeal and *ad hoc*. Australia saw the explosion in infection rates in the IDU communities in New York and Edinburgh early in the epidemic, it saw the confrontational politics between authorities and the gay community in San Francisco, and had the opportunity to shape policy that would prevent an epidemic, not manage an established one.

There is evidence that the Australian National HIV/AIDS Strategy has been comparatively successful. In 1983, one year after the diagnosis of its first AIDS case, Australia ranked fourth among developed countries in terms of AIDS cases per capita (Wodak 1995); by 1991 it had slipped to sixth (and subsequently lower), being overtaken by Spain and Italy where infection rates in the IDU community had soared. Analysis of world-wide government responses to the epidemic (Commonwealth Department of Community Services and Health 1986) indicates that Australia has acted in advance of other countries at a co-ordinated national level, being the first country to screen blood supplies, for example. The national evaluation of the effectiveness of the strategy (Commonwealth Department of Community Services and Health 1992) was able to conclude on the evidence that the epidemic had stabilised in the country and remained confined to men who had sex with men. Such was the confidence in the first strategy, which had been in place until

1992, that it was endorsed almost unchanged for a further three years in 1993.

The success of this policy, and its particular appropriateness in relation to young people, depended on the critical resolution of an early conflict about ownership of the epidemic (Palmer and Short 1994). In 1984, Australia established as a crisis measure two national advisory committees, one from the medical establishment and the other made up of community representatives, that had different and opposing agendas as to how the epidemic should be contained. The debate about controlling the disease by testing and so labelling members of the alleged risk groups, with its attendant inevitable discrimination, had been given an airing already in the United States (Katz 1995). In Australia the debate around the strategies of testing and managing – as opposed to community development and education – was concluded early by the Minister for Health, Neal Blewett, opting to support the latter approach (Altman 1992b) and run with the principles of the new public health. Thus the national strategy was based around the principle that, while HIV is not curable, it is preventable through behaviour change and that education and prevention programmes can bring about such change (Commonwealth Department of Community Services Health 1989). To make such programmes effective, the critical principle of harm minimisation had to underpin every strategy.

Harm minimisation is probably the most essential element of policy in relation to young people. It is particularly appropriate as an approach to accommodate the need that adolescents have to rebel against authority and to make their own decisions. It accepts, non-judgementally, the current prevalent behaviours and seeks to develop short-term and immediate strategies that are more likely to be accepted and so have some capacity to minimise the potential for harm in the existing situation. So, in relation to the sexual behaviour of young people, harm minimisation would work in the following way. The majority of community members may feel that ideally they would prefer young people to abstain from sexual intercourse until they are old enough and mature enough to understand the implications of this behaviour and to manage its consequences. However there is general acceptance that a large number of teenagers, for whatever reasons, are currently having sexual intercourse regularly and will continue to do so. Programmes must then be established that accept the realities of these young people's lives and help them to carry on with an increased degree of safety. This would probably involve provision of non-judgemental explicit information about relative risks involved in different sexual practices, the provision of condoms and of skills development for using them. It does not preclude the possibility of programmes that seek to encourage and support abstinence or the delay of sexual activity running concurrently, but it would acknowledge that such programmes have longer-term goals and limited appeal for some young people.

In the area of IDU, harm minimisation is even more critical and controversial, because in most countries, including Australia, legal sanctions exist against drug use. Endorsement of such an approach under these circumstances pushes the community to tolerate the indulgence and even seemingly the support of behaviours they have chosen to prohibit. While the decriminalisation of such practices or the 'reform' of all those using drugs may be the long-term goals of different segments of the community, a commitment to harm minimisation asks that drug users be supported uncritically to use safely. A hierarchy of risk must be accepted. The worst-case scenario is that users share dirty equipment. If they must share then the preferred option is that they learn to clean equipment consistently and thoroughly, but if they must inject then it is better that they never share equipment. The best-case scenario, of course, is that drug users do not inject at all.

In Australia, harm minimisation in the drug-using area meant a vast increase in methadone programmes and a change in the ideology that governed them, a flourishing of users' groups and peer education and the rapid establishment of needle and syringe exchanges. The needle and syringe exchange programme in Australia is the largest in the world and critical to the maintenance of low HIV infection rates in the country, but is tolerated only as a result of extensive community education and a certain amount of secrecy in its operations. A mobile needle and syringe exchange bus in Melbourne had to be abolished in 1991 because, despite the fact that it was doing more exchanges than any other outlet, the community found it hard to tolerate the notion of a government-funded service available at such 'excessive' convenience to users who had only to dial for a response. In many instances it has not been possible for needle and syringe exchange programmes to survive at the local level because of resident opposition or police harassment. A well-used local needle and syringe exchange in Melbourne was closed as a result of a small number of vociferous residents objecting to drug users being in the locality. The outcome of this was not to send users to another locality in search of another exchange site, but to drive them to more desperate and less safe means of using locally. Anecdotal stories followed of increased sharing and of users breaking into needle disposal units in parks to obtain syringes. Public health, even at the local level, was thus ill-served by this somewhat short-sighted opposition. Another locality successfully addressed concerns about needle disposal with a community development project to ensure disposal facilities were adequate, well placed, thoroughly publicised and supported (Robinson 1994). Where needle exchanges have survived in Australia they have been well used and have played a critical role in keeping HIV infection rates low (Wodak 1995).

An element of policy that makes a harm minimisation approach possible is the notion of 'arm's length' funding. Those communities and groups most affected by the epidemic and most likely to need to make changes in behaviour and culture to prevent infection are critical players in the development of realistic harm minimisation policies and will have, in many cases, sole responsibility for their implementation. Australia then made the decision that money to be spent on the epidemic had to be given to these organisations along with a fair degree of autonomy to spend it. For example, it became evident in the epidemic that safe-sex messages were less likely to be absorbed and translated into practice by a person who lacked confidence in his or her sexual identity or sometimes had mixed or negative feelings about sexual behaviour (McLeod and Nott 1994; Ross 1990). Nevertheless, a government could not be seen to run 'coming out' groups to build the self-esteem of gay teenagers, or to publish safe-sex brochures for gay youth that were couched in the vernacular rather than the clinical, but less communicative, formal language of health and disease. Eroticised brochures with titles like 'Hot tips for hard cocks' and 'Keeping it up', with their more obvious appeal to the relevant quarters, were not produced directly by government funding, but were part of the output of gay organisations whose funding largely came from the government. This type of indirect funding gives organisations more control over the precise focusing of interventions, and removes direct 'blame', with its attendant electoral damage, from the government doorstep.

Nevertheless, such policies can become a matter of public anxiety, as with the mobile needle and syringe exchange, and controls must be exercised. The delicate balance of responsibility and disowning requires constant maintenance and indeed came unstuck in one famous incident that relates specifically to young people. Fears around an increasing HIV infection rate among young men in Victoria who were newly exploring their sexuality prompted the develop-ment of a poster of two young men kissing with a rubric of the 'it's fine to do it but do it safely' variety. This advertisement was to appear in the mainstream press and had to be withdrawn following public outcry about the recruitment of impressionable young men to gay pursuits and under government patronage (McKenzie *et al.* 1992). More angry letters were received by the Minister for Health on this one issue than on any other in Victorian history. But for the most part, arm's length funding is generally particularly successful for services wishing to meet the needs of young people, supply them with condoms or use sexual-health funding to give them food and shelter where these necessities are critical precursors to addressing sexual-health concerns.

A final critical element of good policy that has been characteristic of the Australian experience is a focus on risk behaviours rather than on risk groups. This, more than any other principle, has marked a move away from older disease-control strategies with their focus on the quarantine of individuals and the attendant surveillance, naming and blaming. It has also closed the loophole through which member-ship of 'the general community' (as opposed to minority 'risk groups') can be seen to confer immunity on so-called normal people. It has worked powerfully against the 'them and us' mentality, which can be seen to remove particular entitlements from rejected groups and open the way for discrimination. A policy focusing on risk behaviours does so on the assumption that any person can engage in them at some time or other and is entitled to information to prepare for this possibility. For young people this is of particular importance in relation to their sexual well-being as it is all too easy for peer opinion and peer pressure to result in them excluding themselves aggressively from particular rejected groups. Young people strug-gling to work out a sexual identity or those engaging in casual experimental drug use or in opportunistic sex work need to be able to access information that is not targeted to imply their exclusion. Good policy makes this distinction clear. The refusal to name and blame particular groups and the use of non-judgemental language to describe policy approaches are the primary ways for governments to model a sound approach to HIV/AIDS and work powerfully towards creating a public climate in which it is understood that discrimination will not be readily tolerated.

While it is clear that policy at a national level can have a major impact on the sexual health of young people, they are perhaps more directly influenced by local or institutional policies that have more of a direct or immediate bearing on their daily lives. These policies can be those of schools, of health services, of institutions such as churches and clubs to which they belong, and of services, such as those dealing with housing and employment, that may be essential to their survival. These policies are inevitably influenced and, to some extent, legally determined by government policies and benefit by inclusion of the same critical elements previously discussed. However, there are two additional aspects of this more local policy that are important for young people. These are the extent to which services are made accessible to young people, and the extent to which their confidentiality can be ensured. In most instances they are inextricably linked, the assurance of confidentiality being an essential precursor to service accessibility (Youth Policy Development Council 1987; National Health and Medical Research Council 1992).

CONFIDENTIALITY AND SERVICE ACCESSIBILITY

Sarah goes to the family doctor to discuss contraception, and finds later that her mother has been asked by the doctor to have a word with her. Bradley seeks treatment for an STD at the local health service and finds later that his pathology results, which were negative in any case, were left lying at the reception desk after delivery and were spotted by his girlfriend's father. Kerry goes to a group session for exploring sexual orientation and finds that it is held in a room with a glass wall facing into a busy corridor. Lisa, who is 15, needs the morning-after pill urgently but is worried about what it will cost and cannot get medical attention without having the family health-care card in her possession. Jack would like to know how to use condoms properly but doesn't know whom he can ask without getting a lecture about having sex, or risking someone spreading gossip about him. Cathy is the receptionist at a local medical clinic and finds out there is a boy who is HIV positive in the local youth group her daughter attends; what should she do? For many young people getting help to manage their sexual health is a minefield and policies that are known and understood to guarantee confidentiality can be the most essential key to the maze.

Services and institutions that deal with young people need to be able to gain their trust if they are going to have any impact on their sexual health. The accessibility of a service for young people will often directly relate to its capacity to show that systems are in place to ensure the protection of confidentiality and that the culture of the organisation is committed to this end. Policy is not the only way of ensuring this happens, but it is a critical part of informing young people in advance that they can trust that their business with a particular service will not be inappropriately recorded or divulged. This issue is of primary importance to young people in rural communities (Omelczuk *et al.* 1991) where the levels of community surveillance are higher and the services more interwoven with those of other family members.

Tied in with issues of confidentiality for young people is the issue of contact tracing. The tracing of previous and present sexual partners following an STD diagnosis is extremely important both to enable the individual to access treatment if necessary and to protect others from further transmission of the disease. However, fear of over-zealous and punitive action on this issue from health services can be enough to discourage young people from presenting for treatment. A health service needs a policy for achieving balance between confidentiality and public-health responsibilities that can reassure potential clients that they will not lose control of the situation. In contact tracing, the primary ethical responsibility lies with the infected individual and in most instances they will undertake this task voluntarily. Health services need to have the means to encourage and support young people to do this. They may have cards that can be given to contacts unobtrusively and anonymously, they may offer a service to contact nominated people if the client feels it would be a better way to proceed. Services cannot develop a policy that mandates disclosure of names and addresses of past sexual partners for follow-up unless they wish to be without clients altogether, but they can do much to encourage young people to fulfil this responsibility if they do so without pressure.

Individual health or youth services can develop policies in other areas that also influence their acceptability to young people. Hours of opening can be determined to accommodate the usual commitments of young people. Good universal infection-control procedures can be put in place to ensure there is no need for discriminatory treatment of infected individuals. Distribution of condoms and syringes without question, and the provision of appropriate easy-to-understand information that does not make young people feel patronised or judged, are also matters for policy decisions. Staff training to implement such policies effectively and the involvement of young people themselves in making and sustaining policies are also important in creating accessible and user-friendly services

DISCRIMINATION

Discrimination can be discouraged and even prevented by official policies and the laws that strengthen them. Discrimination is the offering of less favourable treatment and access to services to a person as a result of an attribute or perceived attribute that is believed to make them less worthy. It has a history as long as the history of human society and, in particular, the use of discriminatory treatment as a punishment for sexual misdemeanours is a time-honoured tactic for social control. Women are all too familiar with the operations of the discriminatory double standard around sexual morality. It was for many years enthroned in British law in the notorious nineteenth-century Defence of the Realm Act, regulation 40d, which imposed penalties and forcible treatment on women, but not on men, for spreading sexually transmissible diseases.

Lesser standards of obstetric care provided for unmarried mothers have, right into the mid-twentieth century, been one of the major means by which these women have been encouraged to repent their sins. A British midwife describes these practices in Newcastle in the UK in the 1920s:

> There was a terrible, terrible prejudice about that kind of thing. A terrible stigma.... I do remember that the mothers were not allowed anything to ease their pain, and if they had stitches – well, they just had stitches. I think they'd have done forceps without an anaesthetic. Usually it was done under a general anaesthetic – it was ordinary chloroform or ether for them.
>
> (Leap and Hunter 1993: 114)

Homosexuals have a similar history of rejection and punishment, having experienced the full force of legal sanctions in many societies as well as the demeaning nineteenth- and early twentieth-century pathologisation of their 'condition' (see, for example, Neustatter 1954) to ensure that as sick people certain restrictions would be inevitable. Homosexuality was not in fact removed from official definition as a mental illness in the USA and UK until the mid-1970s (Weeks 1985). In many countries, some aspects of homosexual behaviour remain illegal today. In Britain, where there was a hotly contested attempt in 1994 to lower the legal age of consent for homosexual (anal) intercourse from 21 to 16 (bringing it in line with heterosexual (vaginal) intercourse), 18 was the lowest age that could be achieved (Porter and Hall 1995). In Tasmania, Australia, today the legal age for consent to heterosexual (vaginal) intercourse is 16 years, but it is 21 years for homosexual (anal) intercourse. These examples offer an interesting parallel to HIV-based discrimination because in each of these cases the discrimination that ensues can be constructed as appropriate, given that by their own actions the subjects of such discrimination have brought it upon themselves. Unlike discrimination on the basis of race, appearance or age, for example, which can be seen to be attributes over which a person has no control, discrimination arising out of perceived sexual transgression can be seen as 'a legitimate extension of a punishment already assigned' (Wellings 1994). Those exercising the discrimination therefore can be seen as agents of social control maintaining universally approved moral standards. The establishment of an accepted constellation of risk groups, such as prostitutes, male homosexuals, IV drug users, or promiscuous young people, in which people are identified by their offending behaviours, has fed into this process. The persistent public need to discover how HIV-infected people got the disease and create a hierarchy of blame ('innocent victims', with its implied 'guilty victims') is further evidence of this way of thinking.

Discrimination against HIV-infected people, or those perceived to be potentially infected as a result of their membership of a risk group, has two major sources (Des Jarlais *et al.* 1985; Herek 1984). The first arises out of the moral beliefs already discussed and works through the conviction that these people have done the wrong thing and so have forfeited their right to equal participation in society. The second arises out of fear of infection and has as its argument that, while no offence is intended to the individuals involved, society cannot allow them full participation because it simply cannot risk them spreading the infection further. As there are no circumstances in the case of HIV in which isolating the infected individual is the only, or even the best, form of prevention, this belief arises out of misinformation about the nature and likelihood of transmission. It may then seem obvious that information and education can make a considerable impact on this form of discrimination. Education, one of the major strategies available to address discrimination, will be discussed in Chapter 7.

The discrimination issue has created enormous ethical challenges, some of particular relevance to young people. Debate is particularly lively in relation to universities managing HIV-infected students in health-related areas, where their inexperience or lack of understanding may be more likely to lead to breaches of infection control or other accidents with serious consequences. The law has little clarity to offer about this issue, although anti-discrimination laws allow appropriate discrimination where it can be seen as essential to public safety. The Centre for Disease Control in the United States has advocated that certain procedures be identified as 'exposure prone', therefore requiring that participants in such procedures disclose their HIV or Hepatitis B status. Consensus has never been reached on what these procedures might be. In most cases at present it has been deemed that the infected student has an ethical obligation to withdraw from practices and procedures that he or she judges to be risky, with universities pulling back from the dubious and expensive practice of requiring all students to submit to regular testing. It remains to be seen whether institutions can so adapt essential course requirements and teaching environments to ensure that HIV-infected students can still gain these professional qualifications, and whether society will continue to allow them to practise on such terms. This is a policy area that can be expected to have some consequences for infected young people in the future.

Policy clearly has a critical role to play in addressing HIV-related discrimination, as does the law. Herek and Glunt (1995) suggest three ways in which government policy can address and minimise discrimination. These are the protection of the confidentiality of the HIV status of individuals, the actual legal prohibition of HIV-related discrimination, and public education efforts to reduce unwarranted fears of infection. The issues also relate to policy at a local level. A policy at the very least must require the adoption of procedures, particularly in relation to infection control, that remove the necessity for an individual's HIV status to be known as a means of preventing infection. This relatively simple policy provision in any institution dealing with young people can cut powerfully across arguments to withhold services from those perceived to be at risk. Policy can state clearly that discrimination on the basis of HIV status is not permitted among those bound by its provisions. Indeed, policies that fail to do so can give rise to the institutionalisation of discriminatory practices that can mask and normalise the prejudice of individuals within the organisation.

Those young people likely to experience HIV-related discrimination will almost inevitably be facing discrimination in other ways – for being gay, using drugs intravenously, being homeless, engaging in opportunistic sex work, having haemophilia – they may also face discrimination and its attendant powerlessness simply for being young. Schools and youth services need policies that speak out powerfully against discrimination and offer a proactive advocacy role in gaining for young people the access to treatment services, housing and employment.

Sound policies have the capacity to put in place systems that both ensure that HIV is addressed appropriately and that young people are treated with dignity and equality. They can also assist in loosening the knot between public-health considerations and moral concerns, assisting each to be regarded for what it is. The WHO Forty-First World Health Assembly in May 1988 urged all member states involved in devising and carrying out national HIV-prevention programmes to be mindful of the following exhortations:

1 to foster a spirit of understanding and compassion for HIV-infected people and people with AIDS through information, education and social support programmes;
2 to protect the human rights and dignity of HIV-infected people and people with AIDS, and of members of population groups, and to avoid discriminatory action against them in the provision of services, employment and travel.

It is an important call to nations to ensure such protection is afforded to its citizens and provides a public global criticism of those nations who do not comply. However good policy must arise at a national level with laws that support it, reflecting public consensus on how the issue should be addressed. It is then of great importance that the policy development process within this established framework is replicated over and over again in each institution and organisation to develop the understanding and ownership that are critical for making a policy live and operational.

7 Preventing STDs through education

SUFFICIENTLY FULL FOR THE PURPOSE

As children enter puberty and begin the task of incorporating their emergent sexual selves into their development towards adulthood, they come increasingly 'on line' to receive the messages that any given society is putting out about the dangers of sexuality. Even the most rigid of regimes that strenuously protects the young from worldly knowledge is giving out a message that at this time will be received to help make sense of the nature of sexuality and how it should be regarded. In a very real sense the issue is not whether we, as a society, should be involved in sex education. It is much more important to accept that we are all involved in the conveying of awarenesses in this contentious area and so make some wise decisions about what those messages ideally might be.

The debate about sex education for young people has been a long one, at times bitterly fought. History abounds with pronouncements about the rights and wrongs of such an enterprise, its potential to deflower innocence before its time or to doom to ignorance and danger generations of young people approaching the marriage bed. The time-honoured maxim that 'ignorance is bliss' has never been so seriously contested as it is in relation to sex education for young people.

Historically, sex education was seen to be predominantly moral in its intent, the challenge being how to get young people to do what parents, church or state want while giving them as little potentially dangerous information as possible. Central to the debate has been the concept of young people as both romantically innocent and hedonistically determined to put such instruction to the wrong uses. A booklet, *The House Not Made With Hands* by Mrs E. Josephine Bamford, popularly distributed to adolescent girls in Australia in the 1930s through to the 1950s, illustrates this approach. In a series of 'Talks' to 'older girls', sexuality is equated directly with motherhood, which is 'God's wondrous plan', but is overlaid with heavy religious responsibilities. After considerable attention, literally, to the birds and the bees, there is a rather obscure reference to 'muscular contractions', a prayer, and then a fairly spectacular slippage to the not too specific 'miracle of birth'. These rather opaque details were in fact extremely liberal for the time and were added in to a second more explicit version of an earlier edition after the author received many letters from young women who found adapting the birds and bees to human behaviour a bit difficult to manage unassisted. Despite this, probably unassuaged, anxiety from the readership, the introduction to the book by J. Horace Downing MBBS MSc claims with the highest authority that the information contained therein is 'Sufficiently full for the purpose' (Bamford 1935).

Sex education material for boys from the same era relied a little less on exhortations to responsible manhood, perhaps fearing the target audience to be more intrinsically wayward, and concentrated on physical dangers, most frequently those arising out of masturbation and, less often, STDs. This trend continued most notably in the male-oriented information for the troops in both world wars.

Nevertheless, the opportunity to use health imperatives as the basis for providing information about sexual matters to young people is a relatively new one, arising in the late nineteenth and early twentieth century. The increased public belief in the value of science and the ascendancy of scientific medicine also allowed health enhancement to develop as a moral position. Things now done for 'your own good' became much more likely to be directed towards saving your body than to saving your soul (Foucault 1973). HIV/AIDS has provided the additional incentive of a deadly and incurable disease in an era when medicine had effectively removed the scourges of syphilis and gonorrhoea. Health-based messages have dominated the discourse around sex education for young people for several decades, with the advent of HIV/AIDS withering the final possibility of taking an exclusively moral approach and holding ground.

With the decline in the influence of the church in Western society (although schools and parents may still be powerful upholders of religious beliefs), the primary agents for bringing about change in the sexual behaviour of young people are parents, the peer group, the media and the schools. It is the competing and often contradictory nature of these players that can explain, as much as the well-accepted crisis in the hormones, some of the confusion young people experience today in decision making in their sexual lives.

ROLE OF PARENTS

Parents probably experience the most concern over the transformation of their children into sexually aware young people. Fears for their physical and emotional safety can combine powerfully with grief and regret for the loss of the child and of the relatively straightforward control of earlier parenting. These worries are most acute at a time when the child is moving away from the family unit to interact more potently with the peer group, and when the cognitive development of the young person increasingly allows him or her to canvass a number of points of view to inform a decision rather than an unquestioning acceptance of the parents' wisdom.

Barriers to parents providing information

All this can make it rather difficult for parents to have a role in sex education and STD prevention, and there are certainly many barriers that work against their involvement. A primary barrier is that of embarrassment for both the parent and the young person. Despite possible participation in the 'free love' ethos of the sixties and seventies, most parents of today would have received messages from their own parents that sex was essentially embarrassing and would find some of that embarrassment still operative. The evidence of such awkwardness is readily relayed to a young person and communication blocked by its power. Added to this, young people, as they are moving through adolescence, require an increasing amount of privacy. Intrusions into this can contribute to some of the embarrassment felt.

Parents, who are also all too well aware of the plethora of information on the subject coming at adolescents from all sides, can feel that young people must 'know it all' anyway, and have diminished confidence in their own capacity to provide sound or up-to-the-minute information. This may be especially true in the area of condom use where parents, as children of the pill era, may have no experience of them whatsoever. In addition, parents may share with others in the society the fear that giving young people information will provide them with unspoken permission to go out and try it all. An implicit or explicit assumption may be that keeping children relatively ignorant will ensure the more desirable restraint.

But perhaps the most difficult to deal with of all the barriers is the challenge to parents' own values that the questioning or rebellion of the adolescent may provide. These values, dearly held by most adults, are central to the information and advice that parents are in a position to offer. To feel their values rejected as uninteresting and outmoded can be profoundly painful. For all these reasons it can seem that education about sex and STD prevention is difficult for many parents to undertake. Some understandably feel it is better left to schools and health services.

Do parents have any influence at all?

How much influence parents really have is of course a very complex question and one that is beyond the scope of most research to answer. One way of exploring the question has been to ask young people themselves what they feel about it. In a study that explored sources of information about sexuality and sexually transmitted diseases among Australian high-school students (Rosenthal and Smith 1994), parents were cited as a favoured source of information. A high percentage of these young people said that they would trust information they got from their parents more than that obtained from peers and from the media, but also that they found this source of information difficult to access. Most teenagers said they would like more information than they were getting from their parents.

In an earlier study, 150 sexually active young people from diverse backgrounds were asked about the kind of influences their family had on their ideas about sex (Moore 1994). Responses ranged from the feeling that family had no influence at all to claims that parents passed on values that contributed to shaping sexual behaviour, offering guidance and protection in this difficult area. Other more negative claims were also made including parents curtailing their sexual learning by restrictions on freedom and inhibiting young people's moral development by imposing values of their own. A further suggestion was that parents' stricter ideas and values served an important function by offering young people something to rebel against. This more negative role also emerged in an American study by Darling and Hicks (1982), which found that the messages given by parents were generally cautionary, relying on instilling fear of the consequences of sex before marriage, particularly for girls. A study by Moore *et al.* (1986), however, indicates that this approach is not very successful. With the exception of very conservative parents who had successfully passed their values on to their teenage daughters, parental communication and monitoring apparently did little to discourage pre-marital sexual activity.

In order to assess perceived parental, as compared with peer, influence on sexual behaviour, Rosenthal and Moore (1991) asked sexually active 17- to 20-year-olds about the extent to which parents approved of their sexual behaviour, the extent to which parents had discussed sex, including sexual precautions, and the extent to which parents had actually assisted their son or daughter in arranging sexual precautions. The study showed low perceived approval of sexual activity from parents, with young people predictably finding peers more supportive. Similarly there was little discussion of these matters with parents, particularly fathers. Finally there were even lower levels of parents assisting with contraception, such as condom purchase, indicating that this is a very difficult area indeed for most parents. In a separate study, which asked parents how open they were to discuss sexual matters and how frequently this had occurred, there was a markedly discrepant view from that of the young people (Rosenthal and Collis 1996). Almost all parents felt they were available and open to discussion and were effectively addressing the issues – a view not shared by the teenagers themselves.

As long as most parents rely on cautionary messages with an agenda to prevent their adolescents from initiating sexual activity it would appear likely that their helpfulness will be limited. While young people are reinforced in the perception that sex is for loving and committed relationships, they may feel that the series of 'loving and committed' short-term relationships that frequently characterises early sexual behaviour offers them protection against STDs.

What can parents do?

In spite of all this, parents remain an important influence on the developing adolescent and retain an opportunity to play a role in the shaping of his or her sexual world. In recognising that their teenager is becoming a sexual being and that their influence will be less ubiquitous as the child grows, they will have taken an important step towards a more realistic position. It is important that, in reacting to research that suggests limitations on the capacity of parents to influence and intervene, the contribution of parents is not totally devalued.

Parents have already had a major influence on the child's emerging sexuality before adolescence is reached. Being open to discussing issues and answering questions as they arise in childhood does much to establish a role for parents before it becomes complicated by issues of separateness and privacy. Parents who are less open to discussion or who dodge the issue may find that the messages children absorb from this behaviour have an influence that is hard to dispel as time goes by. Parents also have the opportunity to model desirable behaviour in sexual relationships and to encourage sound patterns of decision making which, in themselves, will stand adolescents in good stead at times when the issue cannot be directly discussed with parents.

Parents may not be able to tell young people what to do and expect blind compliance, but they can offer opportunities for independent learning that contribute to safe and responsible behaviour. Leaving information lying around the house to be picked up and read, offering the name or number of a good health service that the teenager can attend independently, making condoms available in the home with other health items such as tampons and toothbrushes, are all ways in which this can be encouraged.

Finding opportunities for discussion that arise spontaneously, after a television programme for example, can overcome the embarrassment involved in bringing up the subject out of the blue. Beginning with one's own experience can remove barriers created by the so-called 'generation gap' and develop the notion that parents' views arise out of their own experiences and are not blindly and unthinkingly applied. Finally, parents are entitled to their own views and values and are entitled to express them to their sons and daughters, but if they attempt to impose these views 'at all costs', they limit the opportunities for young people to develop personal and thought-out moral codes of their own. Expressing a view or giving advice in this context becomes much more likely to lead to a position of mutual respect.

THE ROLE OF PEER EDUCATION

Peer education has been the linchpin of global AIDS prevention education. The development of the Ottawa Charter for Health Promotion (WHO 1986), which coincided with the increasing awareness of the potential AIDS pandemic, promoted a strong awareness of the value of action at a community level and an understanding of the way in which individual health is dependent on community well-being. Peer education was a strategy that embedded education for behaviour change in the fabric of the local community, and was readily seen as the most useful approach for developing countries with limited resources. A world-wide review of evaluations of AIDS prevention programmes between July 1998 and July 1989 concluded that peer involvement in the planning and implementation of such programmes was a valuable way of ensuring positive outcomes (Stoller and Rutherford 1989).

The gay community, which was – at least in Western countries – the first group to experience the full impact of HIV infection, realised early in the epidemic that changes to the culture had to be made and sustained from within if transmission was to be limited. Peer education and peer-based campaigns became the most valued and effective means of promoting behaviour change in this community (O'Donnell and Jackson 1990; Connell and Kippax 1990). Similarly, among IV drug users, peer education offered a means of reaching a community without a well-defined identity. A meta-analysis of 143 peer-based programmes for adolescent drug prevention showed that peer-based programmes were the most effective for all the outcomes measured (Tobler 1986).

The interest in using peer education for STD/AIDS prevention with young people arose readily in this climate, but also because the well-established role of peer influence in adolescent development had already been recognised by health promoters (see, for example, Ajzen and Fishbein 1977; Ajzen and Madden 1986; Irwin and Mill-stein 1986). Peer education in its various forms has been one of the most widely used means of influencing adolescent behaviour in the era of AIDS (Sloane and Zimmer 1993), often in association with other popular culture 'gimmicks', such as temporary tattoos, comics, stickers and swap cards. It is certainly a major approach used with difficult-to-reach young people outside schools, and by clubs (for example, the Scouting Association) and organisations such as young people's health services. While some evaluations exist (Fennell 1993; Richie and Getty 1994; Slap *et al.* 1991), most of these programmes, because of their very localised quality, have not been documented let alone evaluated, so the effectiveness of this approach is largely unmeasured.

The influence of peers in relation to information about sexuality and sexual behaviour has been well documented, however. Studies examining the influence of parents and peers on young people's attitudes (see, for example, Moore and Rosenthal 1991a; Dunne *et al.* 1993a) have indicated that young people feel more comfortable talking to peers rather than parents about sexual behaviour and feel that peers are more likely to approve of their behaviour. Same-sex peers and older siblings, particularly girls, were trusted sources of information for the majority of young people (Rosenthal and Smith 1994). In relation to condom use it has been demonstrated that beliefs about what peers were doing influenced young people's own condom use (Dunne *et al.* 1993a). In a study in which eighty-two young people were asked about outcomes of a peer education programme compared to an adult-led programme, both programmes fared equally well on measures of imparting knowledge (Rickert *et al.* 1991). However, the peer educators were asked more questions than the adults and greater attitude changes appear to have been recorded as a result of this. On balance, the value of shifting peer attitudes to safe-sex practices seems indisputable.

What is peer education?

Peer education in relation to sexuality education for young people can mean many things. Broadly speaking it is a programme of education that is, at least in part, devised and delivered by young people for young people. These young people must also identify with and be part of the particular sub-group with which they are working: for example, members of a youth club, particular school groups, homeless young people in a locality, gay young people. Sometimes the identification can be stretched beyond same-status peers, as in a programme in Australia where medical students return to their old schools to act as peer educators. In all cases, peers are given some specialised training, which includes STD/AIDS prevention knowledge and some understanding of how to impart it. Beyond that, expectations vary enormously.

Four models of peer education for young people that have been discerned from the plethora of programmes in this area are peer influence, peer teaching, peer counselling/facilitating and peer participation (New South Wales Department of Health 1994).

Peer influence relies on developing an improved awareness of health-enhancing behaviours in members of a particular group in the hope that it will permeate the culture and influence behaviour change over time. There are no set expectations of the trained young people beyond what they choose to do for themselves, and no set time frame in which change is measured or expected. This strategy might be used by an outreach worker with transient populations of young people who are hard to reach in any formal way.

Peer teaching involves training a limited number of influential peers to take on a specific teaching role, often in a more formal setting such as a school, with a view to providing education in a more personally relevant way to young people. The education may not vary in content from programmes otherwise delivered by adults, the role of the peer educator being to model and promote desired behaviours. There are usually no expectations of these trained peers beyond what they are expected to deliver in actual education sessions. This model might, for example, be used in a school where older students, rather than teachers, deliver sessions to those slightly younger with a view to making the messages more relevant and appealing.

Peer counselling and facilitating usually require the selection for training of more highly skilled young people who may have the capacity to learn and exercise counselling skills. In reality, peer educators trained for this role are more likely to provide one-to-one education and advice than in-depth counselling. They can also have a powerful influence in providing links between disenfranchised young people and particular services. This model is often used in the gay community to enable young gay people to work with peers who contact services, with a view to bringing them into more formal education programmes also run by peers.

Peer participation programmes involve young people in the planning and devising of a programme from the outset. They may also be trained to act as educators, facilitators and so on as part of the programme, or the programme may subsequently be run by others according to the peer-devised guidelines. Rather than being true peer education, this can probably more appropriately be seen as a strategy for devising a sound education programme for young people. Many community-based organisations such as local health services, youth housing networks and youth clubs would, as a matter of course, devise all programmes for young people in this way.

The comparative value of each of these models is difficult to comment on as each has its uses in particular circumstances. Comparative evaluations have not been undertaken, and measurements of the effectiveness of one programme do not necessarily apply to another in this area. Peer education programmes often suffer from a lack of clarity about the expectations of trained peers or the proposed outcomes. It has often been said that the only people who really benefit from peer education programmes are the peer educators themselves. While this benefit for the educators should not be disregarded, such a lack of clarity can lead to frustrations and disappointment that run counter to the positive outcomes these programmes can offer. The unquestioning adoption of peer-based sexuality education as most appropriate for young people appears to be founded on the very real perceptions of the potential of peer pressures and peer norms to subvert health-enhancing behaviours. It is important that its value is set against research that indicates some distrust of peer sources compared with those more official sources that, admittedly, are less accessible to young people (Abraham *et al.* 1991; Rosenthal and Smith 1994). When it comes to placing faith in just one approach, peer education may be as limited as any other. Nevertheless, in conjunction with other forms of sexuality education its role can be a powerful one and it may well be the only available means of working with hard-to-reach young people.

For this reason it is important that peer education programmes get more attention from researchers and evaluators. It is also important that the use of peer education is managed well so that it has the maximum opportunity to fulfil its goals. Guidelines prepared to assist the development of this kind of education (see, for example, New South Wales Department of Health 1994) agree on a number of important considerations. Peer education programmes do need to be well planned, and this should usually be with the involvement of the young people themselves who are supported to set realistic objectives that they believe to be worth while. There must be some form of ongoing support for the trained peers, support that they can access readily as they need it. Finally there must be a serious recognition of the contribution of the young people, sometimes with some form of payment being involved. Within such guidelines it would appear that peer education has a valuable contribution to make to STD prevention education for young people.

OPPORTUNISTIC HEALTH PROMOTION

Much has been written on the difficulty of getting adolescents to personalise the threat of HIV/AIDS or other STDs (Moore and Rosenthal 1991b; Wilders and MacCallum 1990) when the 'can't happen to me' ethos is so prevalent (see Chapter 5). In this context the opportunities that arise for one-to-one HIV prevention education when the young person has some cause for fear and concern cannot be overemphasised.

Young people who attend health services for the 'morning-after pill', for an HIV test based on some acknowledgement of risk behaviour, or for treatment for a symptomatic STD are at a particularly receptive point for some prevention education. At this point they are actively engaged in seeking assistance and information. While the distress inherent in the immediate situation might at times work against the value of education given, the potential exists for a one-to-one counselling and educative relationship to be formed (Commonwealth Department of Health, Housing and Community Services 1992).

Education in this situation is not helpful if it takes the form of a lecture or involves criticism of the young person's failure to use protection. A non-judgemental attitude in the health-care provider or counsellor is essential, along with a sense of comfort in discussing explicit sexual behaviours and diverse sexual experiences. If information is presented at this point in a positive and supportive way, it can be seen as tailored directly to the young person's current need and more likely to have an impact than broad education programmes at other times. This sort of health promotion can do much to augment and sharpen the impact of broader education already received.

The trend to provide health-care services of some kind on-site in schools for these reasons is to be applauded. Not only can one-to-one counselling be given in this situation, but also the likelihood of the young person creating such an opportunity is greater if there is the convenience and the protection of privacy that a general-purpose school-based clinic can offer. While evaluations of the impact on behaviour change of school-based clinics in the USA have reported inconsistent findings (Kirby 1992), it would appear valuable for this initiative to continue in the future.

ROLE OF THE MEDIA

The media have an almost inescapable appeal to young people. Grounded as they are in aspects of popular culture and linked to fashion and notions of modernity, their authority can be all-pervasive. As well as using sexuality in exploitative ways, such as is evident in advertising or some pop music, the media can package sexual information in ways that protect the privacy of young people. Information can be gained serendipitously while watching a soap opera, listening to the radio or reading a fashion magazine. The young person does not have to come out and identify as someone who is poorly informed or who needs sexual health advice. They can receive such information and advice without even recognising a need for it.

The use that young people make of media sources in seeking information about sex has been well documented (see Abraham *et al.* 1991; Harris *et al.* 1991; Stancombe 1994). An Australian study (Rosenthal and Smith 1994) found television to be the media source most used by high-school students, with radio also being well used. Magazines were popular but far more with girls than boys.

Media that specifically target young people will understand readily the capacity of sexual advice to sell magazines or create an audience, and such opportunities are not always abused. Many of these teenage magazines have of recent times published articles that offer sound information about sexual health and promote a culture of safe sex. Many have a regularly featured 'doctor' column, which, in contrast to the old agony column dealing with the full gambit of courtship disasters, promotes the importance of medical advice about sexual behaviour and sexual competence. In addition, a whole range of media-based productions such as soap operas, pop songs, and radio talk-backs have at times taken it upon themselves to adopt a safe-sex stand.

However, the popular belief that the media are trend setting, creating and developing new ideas and concepts, pushing the boundaries of the known world, can act to disguise the very real sense in which the media are excessively conservative, following rather than leading, maintaining and promoting the commercially and politically solid status quo. The developing area of cultural studies has increasingly been able to supply the means by which the nature and the power of media messages can be explored, and the confusions that arise out of this contradiction made more explicit.

For example, the way in which the media contribute to the construction of femininity in teenage girls has been widely discussed (Gilbert and Taylor 1991; McRobbie 1991). This is particularly so in reinforcing conventional sex roles and the perpetuation of gender inequalities, to which both soap operas and romantic fiction make no small contribution. Adolescents reading popular magazines are attracted by the way these texts offer to fulfil their fantasies. By reading them and identifying with the ideal teenagers that 'mirror' them from the pages, they learn much about what it is to be normal and socially acceptable, particularly in relation to gender roles (Misson 1994). The implications of these powerful messages for sexuality educators require further exploration, as do the ways they can be used to subvert some of the more dangerous aspects of the process. Girls, for example, are presented as needing to read up on and work hard on relationships, as they are given all the responsibility for making the relationship work. Boys, however, are exempted by popular culture from such responsibilities and allowed a more free-ranging interest in leisure pursuits (Misson 1994). The follow-on from this is all too evident in the power imbalance experienced by young people in relation to sexual behaviour (Kippax *et al.* 1994).

The positives and negatives of media sources specifically as sex-education interventions have been recently explored in relation to sex-based talk-back radio shows (Fahey and Mitchell 1995). This study examined such a programme on a popular teenage radio network in which callers (usually not teenagers themselves) rang up a doctor to ask about both medical and relationship problems relating to sexuality. The study found the programme had several positive features in relation to STD prevention for young people. The first was that the advice of the doctor appeared to be sound and helpful, in most cases suggesting a service from which individual help could be gained and at times even suggesting the kind of questions it might be helpful to ask at such a visit. Second, the use of callers to talk about their own problems helped to personalise what can at times be an impersonal and rather scientific discourse of sex education, so making it more interesting and relevant to young listeners. Finally, a unique capacity to bring discussion of a wide range of sexual matters out of the private and into the public domain while still offering a degree of protection was seen to have positive benefits in the education of young people.

Nevertheless, the use of such programmes as sources of sexuality education for young people was here limited in one very significant respect. By using a methodology based on discourse analysis (Potter and Wetherall 1987) and using the radio programme as text, it was possible to discern that the efforts made by the show's presenter to appear liberal and non-judgemental regardless of the issue were something of a veneer. Without moving into a strictly moralistic or even didactic mode, the presenter exercised a considerable degree of control over the nature of the advice distributed, being able to ensure by a thousand subtle means that it was maintaining a socially acceptable, quite conservative heterosexual status quo. So complex are the operations of this power that it is unrealistic to imagine that even the most discerning of young people could perceive the messages as anything other than confusing. This confusion, because its source is not clearly delineated in the programme, may appear to be the problem of the young people themselves and so represents a hindrance to developing sexual competency. This is a serious limitation on the value of these programmes to health promotion.

It is important that the media, with all their advantages and their intrinsic appeal to young people, are not overlooked as a potential tool for STD prevention education, but it is also important that they are not romanticised. Their primary aim will always be to appeal and entertain rather than to educate, and education will always be very much a by-product of larger forces working to determine media content. Those concerned with education in this area have much to gain by working with the media to improve the quality of the messages wherever possible. An additional approach that can have a powerful educational impact on young people is to engage them in some rudimentary discourse analysis for themselves. Giving them as part of a school programme, for example, some capacity to look below the surface of media messages will develop in them a critical facility that may enable them to put this source to the best use for themselves. This approach, already well accepted as valuable in the teaching of English (Misson 1994), has much to offer sexual health teachers as well.

The explosion of the Internet and the burgeoning capacity of young people in Western countries to access web sites either through their personal computers in the home or through school-based programmes offer an additional opportunity to educate young people. This medium has all the appeal of the popular culture in which it is embedded and an ability to operate as an interactive self-paced learning opportunity that affords young people the same degree of privacy as do the radio talk-back shows. Already programmes have appeared on web sites offering basic information and the possibility of engaging in debate and discussion using e-mail. As a source it will not, of course, always be free of the contaminants of other media sources; programmes put out for young people will have their own agendas as always. But the possibilities it offers for sex educators and other health promotion are limited only at present by community access to the technology. It may well be the health promotion medium of the future.

THE ROLE OF SCHOOLS

For better or worse in Western society at least, a large number of young people get some sort of sex education, however minimal, in schools (Forrest and Silverman 1989). There appears to be a high degree of community support for sex education in schools. The debate about whether church, family or school should have exclusive right to undertake such an enterprise was fizzling out when the advent of AIDS delivered the *coup de grace*. A Gallup Poll in the USA in 1987 indicated that 94 per cent of people believe schools should have an HIV/AIDS prevention programme, and that 80 per cent of parents wish their children to learn about safe sex as an AIDS prevention strategy (cited in Kirby 1992). In Australian research, 85 per cent of students surveyed cited teachers as a useful source of sexual health information and 90 per cent saw school programmes as their major source of information in this area, believing them to be legitimate and reliable (Rosenthal and Smith 1994).

Sex education to a 'captive audience'

Schools appear to be an obvious site for sex education in that the vast majority of young people attend school for some period of time, and that the primary purpose of schools is to educate (Kirby 1992). Both these features create what can be seen to some extent as a 'captive audience' and provide a window of opportunity that does not necessarily occur later when a pressing need arrives. Workers with homeless young people, for example, have commented on the difficulty of finding opportunities for education in this population, regretting opportunities lost when these young people were in school (Mitchell and Rosenthal 1994). In addition, STD prevention programmes in schools offer the possibility of reaching into the community in other ways, such as through parent involvement in programme development and delivery, or the involvement of health-care professionals with the school.

Nevertheless, the concept of sex education in schools carries with it a number of difficulties. First, unlike the family, schools offer no real possibility of tailoring a programme to the individual needs of young people according to their level of sexual awareness and activity. Programmes in schools must be delivered uniformly to all the 16-year-olds or all the 12-year-olds as part of the timetabling. While this can have the advantage of impacting on the whole peer culture in which young people's social lives are conducted, it also has drawbacks. Curriculum must be devised by a centralised process, which may well be consultative and strenuously negotiated, but which offers little capacity to take account of the demands of religion, culture or personal morality in so far as they are diversely represented in school populations. While there is usually some discretionary process for parents to withdraw children from formal sex education programmes, the more currently highly favoured approach of integrating this material across the curriculum makes this difficult. Thus the nature of the content of the programmes can be bitterly contested both at a school council level and at government policy level. The compromises involved in resolving such conflicts can result in a retreat away from the difficult but critical areas where sexual explicitness is required.

This sliding scale of what is permitted, what we can risk teaching young people, is closely linked with a second difficulty of who is willing and available to do the teaching. The category of 'trained sexuality education teacher' is a narrow one indeed, and a more populous category is that of 'teachers who could possibly be conscripted to take it on'. In this latter category are biology teachers, student welfare co-ordinators from a variety of disciplines, physical education teachers, English teachers and home economics teachers to name a few more common ones. The assumption that anyone can teach sexuality as all adults are experts is an erroneous one and assumes both that there is a standard baseline body of knowledge and that all adults can maintain the degree of comfort needed to teach credibly in this notoriously difficult area. Also assumed is that teaching strategies appropriate for more knowledge-based subject can be adapted to an area where challenging values and changing behaviours are primary aims. Teachers have reported strong feelings of inadequacy and lack of both pre-service training and ongoing professional development as barriers to schools developing programmes (Ollis 1995).

In spite of these drawbacks, schools provide a unique opportunity to reach a population of young people with a high degree of interest in sexual issues and behaviour and to work with them in an ongoing way, creating a supportive environment in which a commitment to sexual health is seen as positive. They also offer the opportunity for the wider community to become involved in comprehensive programmes with the promise of extending their reach beyond the classroom. At best, such programmes can be very cost-effective with those already engaged in teaching taking sexual issues on board as opportunities arise. This can only be realistically expected however if adequate resources are available for teacher training and curriculum development.

AIDS prevention or sexuality education?

The need to accommodate all values and views in a single programme has inevitable consequences for what can be taught in a school. The traditional knowledge-based aspects of sex education generally fare well as they are of a piece with the didactic nature of much school teaching and do not require the specialised teaching skills discussed earlier. Science programmes in biology, zoology and human biology can readily absorb lessons on the reproductive organs and their functions or the nature and aetiology of STDs. Epidemiology and population control can be safely dealt with in geography classes and enhance credit for giving some attention to sex education. The plumbing of reproduction, well beloved of the marriage guides of previous decades, has long had a place in school programmes to the point where its inoffensiveness has placed it beyond moral question. The increasing awareness of growing teenage pregnancy rates has permitted an inclusion of contraceptive information, and the advent of HIV/AIDS has allowed, however grudgingly, some attention to safe and unsafe sexual behaviours.

Ehrhardt (1993) suggests that there have been three goals of sex education over the last few years. They are family planning and the prevention of unintended pregnancies, disease prevention, and finally the preparation for a healthy and satisfying sex life. The debate about the content of programmes in schools has generally revolved around this third aim, the other two being placed out of contention as they are seen as falling within the domain of health and well-being. The extent to which messages in schools can be sex-positive and the consequences of encouraging young people to have a positive regard for themselves as sexual beings are issues that remain not only unresolved but in many cases unconsidered. Additional aims that might be included as part of this third goal are the development of an appreciation of sexual diversity (Sears 1992), and an enhanced awareness of the way in which gender inequalities and the operations of power in sexual relationships can be detrimental to young people of both sexes (Patton and Mannison 1995; Peart *et al.* 1995). A comprehensive and effective sexuality education programme must include consideration of these issues. Unfortunately, ideas that challenge conventional views of what is morally acceptable drop readily off the agenda in favour of an information-based, health-related approach.

Nowhere is this issue more evident than in the arguments around the introduction of an appreciation of sexual diversity into general sex education. Partially based on the emphasis on the development of positive identity within the gay community to combat the spread of HIV, the move has at least tenuous links to disease prevention. More importantly it has the potential to liberate young people from the anxiety of confusion about sexual identity and to create a supportive environment in which young people who feel that they may be gay can explore such a possibility safely. However, the justification of disease prevention also works for the opposition who sees this initiative as likely to encourage in the young a wild desire to try out something they would otherwise have had no idea existed, and so lead to further spread of infections.

> Safe sex is vital but I don't believe that youths as young as sixteen need to be taught that anal stimulation...such as licking, is an exciting sexual option.
>
> (Senator John Herron quoted in *The Age* (Melbourne),
> 1 February 1995)

The belief that young people will at once try anything they find out about relates closely to fears of difference (Wille 1995). A persistent belief in the transmissibility of homosexuality and the extent to which young people can be corrupted and doomed to a lifetime of perversion without their initial consent also characterises this discourse.

> Just as the tobacco industry wants more smokers, the gay community wants more gays....[AIDS Council safe-sex advertisements are] unequivocally aimed at recruitment.
>
> (Letter to the *Herald* (Melbourne), 31 July 1990)

There is a sense though in which the implicit heterosexism in schools substantially disadvantages those young people who experience themselves as different, or who actively identify as lesbian and gay (Uribe and Harbeck 1992).

Central to the debate about issues such as this is the long-term conflict between those who believe that repressing the sexual behaviour of young people will reduce its negative consequences, such as STDs, and those who believe that an acceptance of teenage sexuality is the most productive approach, in that it gives young people the information and wherewithal to protect themselves against these negative consequences (Ehrhardt 1993). Whitehead (1994) extends this issue further to ask whether we wish to train young people to take control of their sexual lives from the time that they are likely to become sexually active, or whether we believe that adolescents need time to develop the maturity required for responsible sexual behaviour by a period of adult-enforced protection until their social and biological maturity are better matched. Evidence for the efficacy of either approach is inconclusive.

What works? What doesn't?

Of all the areas in which to carry out evaluation, the assessment of the effectiveness of school-based programmes in changing behaviour must be among the most difficult. While it is possible to establish that most adolescents have a good knowledge base regarding HIV transmission (Anderson and Christenson 1991; Dunne *et al.* 1993a), it is difficult to prove the contribution of school programmes to this knowledge. In fact, the spectacular discrepancy in high levels of knowledge about HIV and poor levels of knowledge about other STDs (Smith *et al.* 1995; Wilders and MacCallum 1990) may indicate that media attention to HIV in particular is as educative as programmes in schools.

This highlights the impossibility of assessing something like risk-taking behaviour, which is so embedded in developmental and social circumstances that the impact of any one thing cannot be determined. The review of the effectiveness of school-based programmes commissioned by the Division of Adolescent and School Health within the Centre for Disease Control in the USA in 1993 (Kirby *et al.* 1994) reported the difficulties of making comparisons between a number of evaluation studies based on different indicators. The resultant study was able to assess comparatively twenty-three studies that met a series of specified criteria and so draw some conclusions in this notoriously difficult field.

Some components of school programmes did not seem to be relevant to either effective or ineffective programmes. Length of programme, the longest being the best, was not an assumption supported by this research. Skills development and practice was another component that was equally present in both effective and ineffective programmes. Two elements of ineffective programmes could be discerned. First, they had a less focused and more broad-based curriculum, and, second, they involved general, rather than specific, decision-making models that sought to teach students how to make good decisions after learning the steps in a given model. Neither of these were seen to achieve the desired end. More importantly, some distinguishing characteristics of effective programmes were isolated. These were:

- a narrow focus on a few specific behavioural goals to reduce sexual risk-taking;
- the use of social learning theory as the basis of a programme (an approach also shown to be effective in relation to other risk-reduction behaviours);

- the provision of basic, accurate risk-related and risk-prevention information through experiential means with a capacity to personalise the information;
- the inclusion of activities to address the power of social and media influences in this area;
- the strengthening of individual and group norms against unprotected sex through the reiteration of clear and appropriate values;
- the use of peer education;
- modelling and practice in communication and negotiation skills.

Also emerging from this study was evidence that school-based programmes did not increase the levels of sexual activity or hasten its onset. This finding was confirmed by Baldo *et al.* (1993), who also found some evidence that such programmes delayed the initiation of sexual activity. Kirby and his colleagues further concluded in his evaluation that there was no evidence that school-based programmes advocating abstinence delayed the onset of sexual activity or reduced teenage pregnancy rates.

It must be made clear that these elements of successful programming emerged only as a result of assessment of particular programmes that were evaluated within very` specific criteria. Frequently the aims of the programmes are so diverse as to make comparative evaluation meaningless. Ehrhardt (1993) refers to an evaluation of differently constructed, more relationship-based programmes in Germany (Schmidt *et al.* 1994), which indicate that young people saw sex as increasingly linked to love and commitment. She also notes the discrepancy between the high rate of teenage pregnancy in the United States and those of other economically and socially comparable countries, such as Canada, France and Sweden, and suggests that school-based programmes with explicit messages consistently reinforced throughout society might be responsible for the lower rates (David 1993; Dryfoos 1985).

By and large, the majority of school-based sex education programmes remain unevaluated, and much of what is favoured, tried and true is valued because it appears to be successful, not because it has been demonstrated to be so by research.

An ideal school-based programme?

As well as those elements identified in the evaluations, there are a number of other factors that may well contribute to maximising the opportunity that exists for sexuality education in schools. While debate rages about the age at which such programmes should start and the content that might be involved, few would argue against the belief that programmes must be age- and experience-appropriate (Ehrhardt and Wasserheit 1992). Placing such programmes in a developmental context and making them age- and gender-specific is likely to make them more focused and appropriate (Ehrhardt 1993). Programmes that adopt an approach based on a social influence model, found already to be successful in programmes to develop other health-enhancing behaviours (Kirby 1992) appear most likely to succeed. These programmes examine the social context in which unsafe behaviours occur and seek to address and engage with the wide range of factors that can cut across and disrupt the best of good intentions. Strategies to recognise and overcome social pressures are the practical basis of this sort of programme.

Dealing with and acknowledging the role of gender and the power relations that affect interactions between men and women (Wyn and Stewart 1991) will create a programme more likely to reflect the reality of most young people's lives. Recognition of the importance of understanding sexual diversity (Ehrhardt 1993; Uribe and Harbeck 1992) will also help such programmes to grapple with central issues for many young people and promote a climate in which discrimination can be minimised. Moving beyond the simple discourse of danger and fear in which much information-based education is persistently embedded will in itself create an opportunity for more informed and responsible sexual decision making by students.

A comprehensive school-wide programme would have links with the wider community; parents would be consulted and may be involved. STD prevention education would be integrated with other curriculum areas, such as English and Social Studies. Such a programme would also recognise the value and proper use of health-care professionals to assist with curriculum development, and support teachers in linking young people into health services. It would value peer education in one form or another to assist with strengthening the social acceptance of healthy sexual behaviour and attitudes. Finally it might operate in an ideal community where the adult norms and values are not in conflict with those we are expecting young people to adopt.

8   Living with sexually transmissible disease

What do I want? A normal life and all the shit that goes with it. Not just the prospect of getting sick and dying. There is this pressing sense of urgency. You have to work it all out before you die. So I work and work on trying to figure life out. But the payoff is that you die.

(Young HIV-infected gay male, quoted in Goggin 1993: 120)

SPECIAL PROBLEMS FOR THE YOUNG

Living with a chronic STD, especially life-threatening HIV infection, is difficult enough to cope with for adults, but for young people the stresses, pains, and conflicts are particularly poignant. Some developmental theory may set this statement in context. The life changes of adolescence include, for most young people, an increase in self-consciousness in its most literal sense. This is the age at which there is more introspection and concern about how one appears to others, and how comfortably one can fit in with the norms and values of the peer group. Coming to terms with sexuality and beginning to experiment with sexual relationships are normal parts of adolescence, and success and confidence in these domains contribute in no small way to self-esteem and self-definition. In addition, planning for the future begins in earnest, and one of the marks of a strong sense of self is the ability to set challenging yet realistic goals. The psychoanalytic theorist, Erik Erikson (1959, 1968), conceives that the establishment of a sense of identity, or coherent sense of self is, in fact, the major life task of adolescence.

What conditions facilitate formation of a secure sense of self? A healthy identity is more likely to develop among young people whose childhood experiences have contributed to good ego strength, that is, children who have experienced secure and reliable relationships, who have been both encouraged and protected in their striving towards independence, and who believe in their own abilities and skills. Further, while some conflict and questioning is seen as part and parcel of identity formation, movement along an identity pathway that places young people too much at odds with prevailing cultural beliefs and norms may make these conflicts too intense for adequate resolution.

For young people who are HIV positive, the 'normal' conflicts and stresses of adolescence and youth are exacerbated many-fold. Although all young people who engage in unsafe drug or sex practices, or are exposed to infected blood products, are at risk, Western world statistics indicate that youthful HIV-positive individuals are currently likely to be homosexual males, intravenous drug users, or haemophiliacs infected through blood transfusions. Each of these groups has special problems to deal with. For gay youth, the 'coming out' experience may have been quite recent, or it may not yet have happened. The anxiety and odd feelings of being 'different' from one's peers, the sense of isolation, and the difficulties of disclosure, all characteristic of the process of committing to gay self-definition, must be re-experienced following HIV diagnosis, as well as, of course, the trauma of coping with a serious and deadly illness. Young drug users, who are likely to have multiple problems and be troubled already, may have difficulties with impulse control and compliance to treatment, and may be living on the streets, and/or selling sex for a living. For young haemophiliacs the issue of seeing oneself as a chronically sick person, with all that entails with respect to identity, must now be overlaid with the need to cope with oneself as an 'infectious' person, infected with yet another stigmatised disease. For each of these groups, the particularly important adolescent tasks of coming to terms with one's body and sexuality, experimenting sexually, developing close relationships, making life plans, and being able to face the future with confidence and energy are severely jeopardised by their diagnosis, even if their symptom-free period lasts many years.

The road to successful coping with HIV diagnosis, and eventually with full-blown AIDS, can be an agonisingly difficult one to follow for young people who might have rightfully expected their life's journeys to be longer and easier. Coping with a disease for which there is no known cure, that carries such social stigma and follows an uncertain and ill-understood course is likely to require not only good ego strength but strong social supports as well. These supports are often more limited for young people. Adolescents find negotiating health-care services difficult enough, but for HIV-infected youth there are very few services anyway. Some adolescents with HIV infection may come from dysfunctional families, or be estranged from their families, perhaps because of current sexual choices or drug behaviours that have contributed to their disease state. Some may be living on the street, dealing with day-to-day survival issues. Reulbach (1991) discusses the problems of counselling chemically dependent HIV-positive adolescents who resist involvement in the support that is available and show poor compliance with treatment. He argues that health workers must first address the chemical dependency (difficult enough in itself) before attempting to help the adolescent work through the expected medical and psychosocial tasks associated with HIV disease.

For the rest of this chapter we shall consider in more detail responses to the diagnosis of HIV and other STDs. Most research in this area has centred on HIV – that is, coping with the symptom-free post-diagnosis period and later with AIDS itself. For this reason, most of the discussion in this chapter is about AIDS-related issues. However, although the other STDs mostly have less serious consequences, they too may require psychological readjustments and lifestyle adaptations. Some discussion of the limited research available on these responses occurs later in the chapter. Much of the research in these areas has not separated adolescent from adult issues, but we shall highlight special youth concerns where that is possible.

RESPONSES TO A DIAGNOSIS OF HIV/AIDS

The doctor was very compassionate, saying that this was probably the worst news I had ever received, and he was right. All of my mental preparation was insufficient to thwart the tidal wave of emotion that swept over me as I received what, at the time, I regarded as a death sentence.

(Ferrara 1984: 128)

When AIDS first became known in the Western world, the focus of diagnosis was on those with end-stage AIDS, that is, those already showing symptoms, usually of a severe nature. Many of these individuals died within a short time of initial diagnosis. As HIV screening became possible and more freely available, the focus shifted towards diagnosis and counselling of those infected with HIV, whether showing symptoms or not (Grant and Anns 1988). This is not to underestimate the needs of those with end-stage AIDS, but to recognise the large number of individuals so infected and the huge range of needs characterising this group, varying as they do in both physical and psychological, primary and secondary, symptoms. Although many young people world-wide are HIV positive, their likelihood of having full-blown AIDS is quite low, unless they have been infected through mother–infant transmission. (See Chapter 1 for statistics on prevalence rates.)

Clinics in various cities and countries now conduct screening blood tests for HIV, and some also provide pre- and post-test counselling (mandatory in some countries). The number of people seeking HIV testing through clinics, hospitals and their local doctors has increased dramatically. Whereas once those already symptomatic, or gay men who believed themselves to be at high risk because of unsafe practices, were virtually the only people seeking testing, there is now a greater tendency for heterosexuals to undergo screening. One trend noted among young people is for couples to both have tests before making the commitment to monogamy and condomless sex (Moore and Rosenthal 1992b). For example:

Would you ever have sex without a condom?

Depends on what you know about the person. After you have been having sex with a person you know them properly. You might even say 'how about we both go and have a test?' to make sure. *(16-year-old male)*

Grant and Anns (1988) have described responses to diagnosis arising from clients, mainly gay men, at the Albion Street Clinic in Sydney, Australia. They note that usually, for low-risk clients, a negative result simply allays concerns that have been felt about a history of unsafe practices, or even a single 'slip-up'. However some clients disbelieve their negative results. These researchers suggest that this is often associated with personality disorder, such as excessive guilt, generalised anxiety, hypochondriasis, and the like. Other writers have discussed a syndrome designated 'the worried well', which may relate to guilt about past sexual habits, or be symptomatic of obsessive compulsive disorder or hypochondriasis (Faulstich 1987).

For a positive diagnosis, however, there are many questions to be faced, such as 'Will I get AIDS? What do my symptoms mean? Why have I become ill? Will I be able to function tomorrow? Will I be able to live with dignity? Will I be able to beat AIDS? Will I be able to die with dignity?' (Weitz 1989). Common short-term responses to an antibody-positive diagnosis are shock, anger, sexual dysfunction and depression. Shock can be expressed in a range of different ways, from short-term regression into immobility – an almost catatonic state in which there is an inability to act or think in any coherent manner – to seemingly casual acceptance typified by comments like 'I thought I would be. . . . No I have no questions, thank you' (Grant and Anns 1988: 73). These reactions are usually short-lived so that the client moves quickly to anger, depression, or some other intense emotional state reflecting the seriousness of his or her diagnosis. Ross *et al.* (1989) studied the case notes of 153 patients informed of their HIV antibody-positive status after testing at an AIDS clinic in Adelaide. They record that, among these clients, initial responses of calm, indifferent denial or the insistency on mistaken diagnosis (as frequently seen in cancer patients) were rarely exhibited. More common was anger, often exacerbated in gay men by the realisation that one has become part of yet another minority, stigmatised group.

Anger is interpreted by Grant and Anns as a healthy reaction to a positive result. It can be directed in a variety of ways, such as at the person considered the carrier of the infection, the situation that led to the infection, healthy people, or the perceived apathy of society. Sometimes the anger is directed at the health worker who reports the bad news, suggests lifestyle modifications, and cannot offer a cure.

High levels of anxiety may be expressed about the practicalities of the situation. There are so many new challenges and decisions to be made that such anxiety can be overwhelming in the early days after diagnosis. Problems to be coped with include: whom to tell; financial, work and family commitments; finding out about the course of the disease; and worry about how long it will take for symptoms to emerge. Sexual dysfunction is common, with recently diagnosed HIV clients having little interest in sex, often feeling dirty, contaminated and expressing low self-worth.

Depression may be a short-term and a long-term response to diagnosis. In the short term, many clients, both younger and older, develop reactive depression, showing apathy, little interest in future goals, and lack of energy and interest in life. The normal planning for the future that is part of the task of youth – interest in careers, relationships, the development of a satisfactory and comfortable lifestyle – may seem futile under the weight of the heavy burden of HIV diagnosis. There may be a withdrawal from social interaction as in the following case example:

Mr. B., a 29-year-old homosexual man, presented as a detached, quiet and defensive individual who appeared to have accepted his HIV antibody-positive status. He was, however, burdened with the fear of being identified as antibody positive to others and his anger over the stigma associated with it. Mr. B. isolated himself from former friends by moving to a boarding house to be alone. Clinical depression with vegetative features was apparent, and he was fearful of losing his job if his antibody-positive status became known.

(Ross *et al.* 1988: 98)

Ross and his colleagues indicate that part of this social withdrawal may include a 'return to the closet' for gay men, as a kind of guilt-induced punishing reaction stemming from internalised (presumably unconscious) homophobia.

COPING WITH HIV ON A LONG-TERM BASIS

Grant and Anns believe that most clients work through some or all of these initial reactions and come to the point of expressing a need for counselling and information to help them cope with the future. Some of the issues commonly addressed are existential and spiritual concerns, relationship issues and 'unfinished business' from the past.

Facing the possibility of death for many means questioning the meaning of life in general, their own life in particular, and making decisions about how one's remaining life should be lived. For some, perceived futility, anger, and/or inability to change because of weak ego functioning mean that the self-destructive lifestyle that sometimes precedes the diagnosis is continued, or may be exacerbated with increased alcohol or drug intake. Others make conscious decisions to make positive lifestyle changes, while others begin a disengagement process from life, withdrawing from friends, family, social and work commitments. Withdrawal from relationships may in part be non-voluntary, as being HIV positive places a great strain on relationships, particularly with sexual partners. Some couples cope with this strain, even strengthening their relationship as a consequence of 'weathering the storm'. Relationships that have not involved good communication patterns, or that are characterised by unresolved conflicts, are far less likely to survive (Grant and Anns 1988).

The issue of being single and HIV positive, more likely to be the case for young people, poses a different set of problems. Young people face fear and rejection if they admit their HIV status to potential sexual partners, or even to new friends. There are reported cases of children being turned away from schools or kindergartens when their HIV status became known in the local community. Laws against discrimination have been enacted in some countries, and privacy laws can protect infected individuals' anonymity, but such laws only go part of the way in changing public attitudes. With respect to sexual relationships, in some countries laws have been changed, adapted or more strongly enforced to discourage HIV-positive individuals from engaging in unprotected sex without disclosing infection status. Of course, relatively safe sex is possible for HIV-positive individuals and their partners if appropriate precautions are taken. Nevertheless the question of when in a new relationship to admit HIV status is a challenging one and sets up an already vulnerable individual for more emotional pain if rejection occurs. Community fear of this currently incurable disease is not surprising, and there are many difficult-to-face current and future lifestyle implications of having an HIV-positive partner. Thus choice of new partners is likely to be severely limited, and the infected person may have to cope with the reality of facing the disease without the comfort of an intimate relationship.

Grant and Anns see coping styles as falling into three categories:

1 those who improve the quality of their lives through adaptive means, such as redefining self-image and emphasising ways to improve health, relationships or spirituality, focusing on living the best way they can and staying as healthy as possible;
2 those who adopt a neurotic, exaggerated or obsessively health/symptom-oriented lifestyle;
3 those who do not cope, and may withdraw, become intractably depressed, and commit or attempt suicide.

The extent to which these coping styles fluctuate or remain stable will depend on clients' pre-existing emotional strengths, their level of support from significant others, and the stage and level of symptomatology of the disease itself. For young people with the possibility of many years of symptom-free HIV status, the encouragement of more positive, life-affirming approaches to the disease by health workers, family and friends, and the community in general, are particularly important.

YOUNG GAY MEN AND HIV

Ross and colleagues argue for five stages of coping, based on their work with homosexual men. Their model of adaptation is based on the grief-work theory of Kubler-Ross, who conceptualised reactions to diagnosis of terminal illness in terms of stages of Denial and Isolation, Anger, Bargaining, Depression and Acceptance (Kubler-Ross 1970, 1987). In Ross's model, Stages 1 and 2 are combined, with anger being a more common reaction than denial, as described previously. Also previously discussed is the Withdrawal/Depression stage, viewed as complicated in some gay men by feelings of guilt and conflict over their homosexuality. Such effects may be more exaggerated in young gay men diagnosed as HIV positive, because of the limited time they have had to accept their homosexuality, incorporate it into a sexual identity, and develop supportive networks. The mood swings and conflicts of identity development, the crises of 'coming out' and learning to deal with a positive diagnosis may be occurring more or less simultaneously for young, HIV-positive gay men.

The Bargaining stage of Kubler-Ross's model is elaborated by Ross and his colleagues into a set of four substages, because of the commonalities and consistencies in responses apparent in their research population. These substages, which parallel to some extent Cass's (1979) model of homosexual identity formation, are described as follows.

(a) Coming out to significant others. This involves disclosing HIV status to selected significant others, individuals who are most likely to be accepting or who have been supportive in the past, such as families and friends. Reactions of such significant others become a sort of 'testing of the water' to broader disclosure. Such sharing also allows some displacement of the stress and anxiety of diagnosis, provides opportunity for others to express their love and support, and begins the possibility of dialogue about fears for the future. The bargaining process involved is of the kind 'If these people whom I trust accept me, then others will too' or 'It can't be so bad' or 'I can share the burden.' For some, this process does lead to nurturing and caring, others need to negotiate acceptance, while others are rejected at this first point of active coping, jeopardising further attempts to martial social support and ultimately develop coping strategies.

(b) Seeking out others in a similar situation, often tentatively at first, is a process that will allow for reinforcement and support from others sharing a common problem. Although difficulties may accompany this substage, such as loss of anonymity and identification with a stigmatised group, seeking out other HIV-positive individuals 'seems to be based on an emerging hope that through an identification with others an unbearable situation can be accepted' (Ross *et al.* 1989: 100).

Particular problems in finding others may occur for young people, who may feel less able to identify with predominant infected groups, which in most Western countries consist of older gay men. Groups like Positive Women have been set up in certain cities to support HIV-positive women, but such groups had great difficulty in forming in their early stages, partly due to stigma and partly because of the small numbers involved. Young infected heterosexuals may feel threatened by predominantly homosexual support groups, and young homosexuals may feel their issues are different from those of an older cohort. Outside major cities, the possibility of finding such support groups is extremely limited, and the threat to anonymity that any available groups pose may loom as a greater problem in small communities. Possibilities of contacting those in similar circumstances are, however, increased by the technology of the Internet, although there is little research available at this point on how such links might assist coping.

(c) Special status. Ross and his colleagues note this substage of Bargaining as common in those individuals previously lacking a strong sense of identity, that is, predominantly young gay men. While some may skip this process, others turn 'alienation into an advantage' by over-identifying with the infected role, seeing themselves as different, special and important on the basis of HIV status. The following case example is given:

> Mr. E., a 24-year-old homosexual man, had always wanted to do something important, and often fell short of his goals. He refused to believe that being antibody-positive made him 'bad', and saw his status as something special. He felt he could contribute to committees and activities designed by gay groups to help fight AIDS, and was not ashamed to tell others he was HIV antibody-positive. His positive approach increased his self-esteem and made him feel more confident, although he still tended to see people in terms of being infected or not.
>
> (Ross *et al.* 1989: 101)

(d) Altruistic behaviour. At this stage there is strong identification with others who live with HIV, which can be marshalled into action such as public support for AIDS awareness, and/or support of others in more advanced stages of the disease. The feelings of community are a positive outcome generated in this stage, but a negative can be burnout and exhaustion possibly leading back to depression and withdrawal.

Kubler-Ross's notions of bargaining were about attempts to look after unfinished business in one's life, to seek some sort of 'truce' with others, oneself or God as a way of trying to stave off the inevitable. In a similar way, the above bargaining substages reflect attempts to lessen the impact of the HIV diagnosis by 'normalising' the disease, integrating it into everyday life, and surrounding oneself with as much support as possible. In these ways, the bargaining process is an adaptive one, but as with the Kubler-Ross stages of facing death, it only goes so far. Normalisation is healthy and adaptive for a time, and in the case of HIV this could be a very long time, given the lead time between infection and symptom production. Eventually a healthy adjustment is thought to involve 'acceptance', that is, acceptance of the disease and the limitations it will place on lifestyle as symptoms increase, and finally acceptance of death as the inevitable outcome. Not all those living with HIV/AIDS will reach this stage of acceptance, or, as with all the stages, there may be fluidity as individuals regress, move forward and regress again. As 'Sonya' puts it,

> People talk about having a positive attitude and that's fine, but you know some days it just sucks, it's dreadful, it's horrible – I wouldn't wish it on my worst enemy.
>
> (quoted in O'Keefe and Walker 1992: 26)

In another example, 'John' expresses acceptance in a very positive manner. His conclusions about HIV making life better may or may not remain with him as the disease develops further, and could appear Pollyanna-ish. But more importantly his ability to 'confront' and accept, even if temporarily, has obviously led to a better life in the here and now.

> HIV has changed my life for the better. It has made me think about stuff that most of us take for granted. It has made me confront my mortality, something I don't think I would have done for decades yet. It has made me think about my relationships with just about

everyone around me.... It has been a very magical change and
overwhelmingly for the better.

(quoted in O'Keefe and Walker 1992: 70–1)

Further issues

An important issue about psychosocial coping with HIV is that it
cannot be seen in isolation from the symptomatology of the
infection. It can be difficult to distinguish some of the neurological
complications of the disease, such as severe depression, from
psychological responses to it (Buhrich *et al.* 1988). Central nervous
complications of AIDS may impair mental acuity and the ability to
cope with stresses. It is estimated that the prevalence of organic
mental disorders occurring at some time during the course of AIDS
is about 65 per cent (Perry 1990). Both delirium and dementia are
common outcomes of central nervous system dysfunction related to
HIV and of the side effects of drugs used to treat AIDS, especially in
its advanced stages. As a result, the frequency of psychiatric and
neuropsychiatric disorders associated with AIDS is high, not
necessarily or only because of coping and adjustment difficulties
(Holland *et al.* 1992).

Another complication of coping with a diagnosis of HIV is that
individuals who develop it have frequently already lost one or more
friends to the disease, and are suffering from bereavement as well as
trying to cope with their own health problems. Dean *et al.* (1988)
studied over 600 gay men in New York City and noted that, on
average, each could name six men who had died of AIDS. Many
suffered the symptoms of bereavement, such as sleep disturbance
and demoralisation.

Not surprisingly, then, Tross and Hirsch (1988) found that 76 per
cent of the AIDS patients they studied met the criteria for a psychiatric
disorder. Common symptoms were anxious and depressed mood,
anxiety and/or panic disorders, and major depression. A study of
HIV-positive haemophiliacs by Dew *et al.* (1990) showed that those
who exhibited the most distress had a family or personal history of
psychiatric disorder, lower levels of education, low social support,
and had experienced a concurrent loss. Overall, prior psychiatric
disorder predicts poorer adjustment. For example, Holland *et al.*
(1992) note that IV drug users diagnosed as HIV positive frequently
present serious behavioural problems, such as non-compliance with
treatment, and psychological problems that complicate their care,
such as continuing with a drug-addictive lifestyle.

On the other hand, there is the question of whether the asymptomatic period of HIV infection is characterised by the emotional distress and stress-related disruption reported for other periods of HIV infection. Blaney *et al.* (1990), in a study of forty-five asymptomatic HIV-positive gay men and thirteen gay men who tested HIV-negative, showed that emotional distress and stress were elevated in the antibody-positive population, but they more closely resembled non-clinical rather than clinical populations on measures of stress and coping. The authors used these data to stress the importance of emphasising the positive coping potential of those with asymptomatic HIV infection.

COPING WITH HIV AS A YOUNG HAEMOPHILIAC

Haemophilia is an inherited, lifelong, chronic disease caused by a deficiency of a clotting factor in the blood. Bleeding episodes associated with this disease, particularly haemorrhages into the joints, can lead to distress, severe pain, and even death. Treatment of bleeding episodes involves infusion into patients' bloodstreams of concentrated clotting factor, which has been extracted from large amounts of pooled human plasma. Self-infusion techniques, which allow patients to treat bleeding episodes as they happen without having to go to hospital, have led to much-improved lifestyles for haemophiliacs. The problem with this treatment is, however, that viruses can be transmitted in the clotting factor concentrates. Hepatitis B and C have been frequent complications of treatment (Gerety and Barker 1976). In the early days of the AIDS epidemic, the HIV virus was transmitted to a large number of haemophiliacs through blood-product treatments. Nowadays, blood is screened; however, the large number of donors needed to produce clotting factor concentrate, and the lack of 100 per cent accuracy of any screening test, mean that some risk must always be attached to this vulnerable group. In addition, there are now many haemophiliacs world-wide who are HIV positive or have full-blown AIDS. Wicklund and Jackson (1992) estimate that one in every twelve haemophiliacs in the United States already has AIDS. In France, Coles (1989) reports that more than 40 per cent of haemophiliacs are HIV positive.

Several issues exacerbate the already considerable problems of coping with a diagnosis of HIV antibody-positivity for haemophiliacs. As haemophilia is an inherited disease, it is not uncommon for more than one individual in the family to be afflicted and therefore to have also contracted HIV or at least be vulnerable. Guilt in families about inheritance of one disease can be compounded with stigma associated with a further disease about which there is a great deal of community fear and suspicion. Many haemophiliacs view them-selves as 'innocent victims' of the virus in the sense that transmission did not occur through sexual intercourse. They feel anger, not only at having contracted the virus, but also at being associated with groups already stigmatised in society. There is anger too at the medical profession, which can lead to distrust, delaying treatment for bleeding episodes, fear of treatment, and failure to follow their medically prescribed regimen. Quality of life may be further com-promised by such non-compliance.

For young haemophiliacs, self-esteem and self-image may be severely disturbed. These young people may already have restric-tions on their lives, such as inability to participate in certain sports and school activities. Such restrictions limit the avenues through which identity can be defined. Added to this, problems of working through issues of relating to others sexually, already difficult enough for adolescents, are made particularly conflict-ridden by knowledge of HIV status. Fear of rejection may lead to social isolation. Over-protection on the part of parents may further curtail quality of life and opportunity to explore identity possibilities in these young people. At the other extreme, feelings of invulnerability characteristic of some adolescents may lead young HIV-positive haemophiliacs to deny their disease status, with potentially serious consequences for their sexual partners.

WOMEN AND AIDS

It is predicted that by the year 2000 there will be nearly as many women with AIDS as men (WHO 1990). In the UK in 1990, 44 per cent of infected women were aged 24 or younger (Bury 1992). So HIV is clearly a disease of younger, rather than older, women. Such women face special problems, such as lack of a community of support, conflict, misinformation and fear about whether to have children, issues around looking after any children they do have, and fear of abandonment. Springer notes 'Women often stick by their men through HIV infection, illness, and death. Men often abandon their women when they become HIV infected or ill' (Springer 1992: 37).

While gay male groups appear to have marshalled resources to provide a great deal of support for HIV-infected people, women infected through heterosexual practices, IV drug use, or medical interventions have been slower, because perhaps of their initially smaller numbers, to group together. This is changing as numbers increase, but the following quotation expresses the frustration of one infected woman.

What I really wanted was to meet other HIV-positive women I could talk to about my fears about having children – or rather not having children – about sex, relationships and so on. This, however, was not as simple as it might first sound. Trying to locate another positive woman in the London area at that time was about as easy as attempting to find a small needle in a large haystack.

(quoted in Thomson 1992: 136)

Mythologies abound regarding advisability of having children for HIV-infected women, probably because early studies were of women whose pregnancies occurred when they were already quite ill with AIDS symptoms. Four dangers surrounding pregnancy for HIV-positive women have been described by Bury (1992) as follows.

1 The danger of pregnancy accelerating the onset of symptoms or the course of the disease. MacCallum and colleagues in 1988 conducted a study of twenty-eight HIV-positive women who were asymptomatic, and found that pregnancy had no effect on their health or immune systems. Other studies have confirmed these findings (Schoenbaum *et al.* 1988), but it does seem that once the disease is at the stage where the woman's immune system has been reduced in efficiency, pregnancy may cause more rapid progression of symptoms.

2 The danger that HIV infection will affect the outcome of pregnancy. There has been little systematic research on the outcome of pregnancies of mothers who are showing symptoms of AIDS. Studies in Edinburgh and New York suggest drug-using asymptomatic HIV-positive women fare similarly in their pregnancies to uninfected drug-users. Research with women who become HIV positive through heterosexual contact or medical accident, but who have had otherwise healthy lifestyles, do not appear to have been carried out at this stage.

3 The danger of infected mothers transmitting the infection to their babies. The virus can cross the placental barrier as early as 20 weeks into the pregnancy. Bury quotes early studies as suggesting a 50 per cent transmission rate, but notes that these studies were of mothers already showing AIDS symptoms. More recent research indicates a

much lower transmission rate, as low as one in eight. If mothers are asymptomatic and healthy, the rate may be even lower, although there is some suggestion that the time a woman seroconverts (becomes HIV positive) may be a particularly risky period for the developing foetus.

4 The danger of infection to the baby during breast feeding. It is difficult to research this possibility, because it cannot be ascertained whether a baby is HIV positive until about 18 months of age, when the infant begins to manufacture its own antibodies. Until then, the child carries the mother's antibodies. Bury sums up the available data and draws the conclusion that the risk is small, but if safe alternatives to breast feeding are available, they should be utilised.

Clearly, for young HIV-positive women, the issue of whether to have children requires analysis of a great deal of information, and that information is continually being updated by more research. Of course, by becoming pregnant naturally, an infected woman risks the health of her partner, but the level of this risk is also extremely difficult to ascertain. One reality to be faced is of not being able to see one's child grow to maturity, but no one can predict just how long an asymptomatic person will live. The comfort, fulfilment and sense of purpose provided by a child may be longed for in women for whom there is little else to look forward to. Counselling and support services must be sensitive to the conflicting fear, longing, and guilt characteristic of this dilemma.

TACTICS FOR PRESERVING MENTAL HEALTH

Bartlett and Finkbeiner (1991) suggest that seeking as many sources of social support as possible is important for emotional survival, and list family, friends, religion, AIDS-advocacy organisations, support and therapy groups, and mental health professionals as potential sources for such support. 'Taking control' is their second maxim for preserving mental health during the course of the disease, by which they mean developing plans and strategies for dealing with the psychological pain and the physical degeneration of AIDS. Suggestions include breaking down what seem to be overwhelming problems into smaller, more short-term and manageable ones, and dealing with those one at a time so as to attain some sense of mastery over the events of life. Finding ways to relax, 'escape' and forget the disease, even if only for a short time, is another technique for coping, as is giving oneself permission to acknowledge and express the emotions of despair, fear and rage that are bound to surface. Focusing on the positive, however, is seen as the single most important strategy for emotional well-being. An example from 'Jean' illustrates the point:

So how has being HIV-positive changed your day-to-day life?

I guess it has given me a different focus on what my life is . . . being HIV positive has made me more positive about myself and where I'm going. . . . I respect myself more now and I want to hang on to life rather than destroy it.

(quoted in O'Keefe and Walker 1992: 88)

A group calling itself 'Positive Youth' expresses this message in its self-description:

We are a group of young people under 26 who are HIV positive and taking responsibility for our lives. The virus is not a death sentence, it is a reason for us to celebrate living. By supporting each other and running our own group, we are able to care for our health and well-being. Our future is in our hands.

(Flyer for Positive Youth, Melbourne, Australia)

LIVING WITH A SEXUALLY TRANSMISSIBLE DISEASE

Other STDs are generally not life threatening in the same way as HIV/AIDS, but young people who are diagnosed with an STD still require coping strategies, to deal adequately with the treatment regimen and the psychosocial consequences. In the case of non-curable STDs, or those with lasting negative effects like infertility, the task of coping may require adjustments to life plans and disruption to relationships. Social stigma is a major issue for these illnesses, and it may serve to limit rational and effective coping. For example even with curable STDs individuals may delay seeking help, or may not explain to partners that they are infected. They may re-establish a pattern of unprotected intercourse after symptoms have gone, even though for some STDs, disappearance of symptoms does not necessarily mean that the person is uninfected or uninfectious. Compliance with medical treatment may be low because of difficulties that the young person experiences in planning, impulse control, or accepting the authority of the medical profession. There may be feelings of shame, anxiety, depression and despair to deal with, as well as the disease itself.

Analysis of interviews with fourteen women and four men with herpes, mostly recruited from self-help groups, indicated that while the physical symptoms of this disease were often extremely painful and debilitating, for many the worst aspects were emotional (Pyett 1995). As one young woman explained:

> the pain of it, um, is horrible. But it's not a stitch on what it does to your nervous system, emotionally. It's like PMT ten times [worse], you know.
>
> (quoted in Pyett 1995: 4)

Most of this study's participants had experienced shame and guilt about their condition, and felt dirty, isolated and unable to talk to others about it. One woman said she felt like 'a big germ', and another as if she had 'a big H' on her forehead. Fears of infecting others were high and those affected felt sexually undesirable and feared rejection from possible partners because of the stigma associated with herpes.

An article by Reiser (1986), 'Herpes: A physical and moral dilemma', presents further evidence of the perceived stigma associated with STDs. This researcher asked college students how would they go about telling a dating partner if they had been diagnosed with herpes. Also, what would they do if a girlfriend/boyfriend told them he/she had herpes? A significant proportion indicated that they would be unwilling to admit to their diagnosis, and many said that they would terminate a relationship if their partner had herpes. Study participants clearly viewed the issue of telling or being told about herpes as a difficult moral dilemma, one fraught with emotion. One imagines that telling a partner about non-sexual infectious diseases, such as chicken pox or the flu, would elucidate a far lower level of emotional response.

In relation to this point, Rosenthal and Moore in a 1995 study asked students to rate how they would feel if they were diagnosed with a range of different diseases, some of them sexually transmitted, some not (see also Chapter 3). The rating scale comprised fifteen negatively valued adjectives – embarrassed, guilty, worried, angry, unclean, frightened, ashamed, degraded, unlucky, responsible, infectious, open to criticism, limited in your activities, dependent on others, and depressed. Attitudes were more negative toward the STDs, with AIDS attracting the most negative attitudes. The adjectives 'ashamed', 'unclean', and 'degraded' were most strongly associated with the STDs, while 'angry', 'depressed' and 'frightened' were the key descriptors of feelings about the non-sexual diseases. It would not be surprising if the strong emotional responses, particularly that of shame, associated with STDs, led to inappropriate responses to symptoms, as discussed previously.

In fact, having been treated for an STD in the past does not seem to relate to future preventive practice, indicating that young people often do not respond rationally to these diseases. O'Campo *et al.* (1992) studied over 500 women, the large majority under 30, attending for prenatal visits at a large American hospital. Of this sample, 36 per cent reported having had a previous episode of an STD. Results of the study showed no relationship between previous STDs and current STD/HIV preventive practices. The authors concluded that diagnosis and treatment for an STD needs to be supplemented with counselling and information. The study is consistent with one targeting adolescents, in which there was also no evidence that a previous STD led to greater efforts to decrease further exposure to STDs (Fullilove *et al.* 1990).

Perhaps because STDs cover such a wide range of diseases, some readily cured, some chronic, some with relatively minor symptoms, some with symptoms that are severe and/or long lasting, little research on coping with STDs has been carried out. The models and theories that have been put forward to explain coping with disease in general may (or may not) apply to STDs. The fact that we are talking about diseases transmitted sexually and involving symptoms relating to sexual body parts may mean that strategies for coping take on a different flavour. One model that has been put forward to help explain how people deal with disease is Attribution theory (for example, Taylor *et al.* 1984). An example study, of women with breast cancer, showed that behavioural self-blame (the belief that the patient could have prevented the disease through her own actions, such as through not smoking) and characterological self-blame (the patient's belief that she is the sort of person to whom negative things happen) led to different adjustment outcomes. Those who used the former strategy were less likely to perceive themselves as vulnerable to recurrence. They also coped less well with the disease, as assessed by various indices of adjustment (Timko and Janoff-Bulman 1985). Could such a model be applied to individuals with, say, herpes? In the case of this and other STDs, the possibility of blaming one's sexual partner or partners is of course an option. How would this affect adjustment, treatment compliance, feelings of shame, and the like? The options for fruitful research in this area are wide open.

9   Conclusion

HAS ANYTHING CHANGED?

Substantial resources have been allocated to educating young people to adopt safe sexual practices, including national media campaigns, school-based education programmes and other community initiatives. But have the safe-sex messages been effective in persuading young people to change their behaviour? When asked, 'Will AIDS affect how you go about sex in the future?', many 16-year-olds in one of our studies gave replies that reflected a heightened concern about having unprotected intercourse (Moore and Rosenthal 1992b).

Yes, for sure. I would be a lot more sure about precautions and who I was sleeping with, and make sure I know about their past.

Yes, if I was really serious with some guy I would get an AIDS test done and he would get one as well.

I think in the future I wouldn't sleep with anyone without a condom. If I was in a casual relationship it wouldn't bother me using a condom all the time, but if I was in a steady relationship I could quite easily say to them, 'come on, let's go have a blood test'.

Yes, you will be more cautious. You don't just jump in the sack with any old guy.

I will always be careful about it. Twenty years ago you didn't have to worry about it, but nowadays with AIDS, you have to worry.

Yes, definitely. It will affect the people that you sleep with and when you sleep with them in your relationship, and wearing condoms. I mean in the old days if they were on the pill you would probably just leave it at that, but you can't do that these days, you have to use condoms as well.

All of the above young people have thought through some reasonable (although not necessarily perfect) strategy for safer behaviour, whether it be condom use, selection of partner, or blood tests for HIV infection. It was encouraging that some of these young people were also aware that the risks resulting from unprotected intercourse extended to sexually transmitted diseases other than HIV and AIDS.

> I think it depends on how bad it gets. But it's not just AIDS you have to watch out for – it's hepatitis B and gonorrhoea and syphilis, and I have heard that they are incurable now too.

The quotations reflect the research findings that young people's ideas about sexual practice have changed. Safe sex has now achieved the status of a cultural norm and is recognised by most young people as the right and proper approach to sex, whatever the barriers may be to operationalising this ideal. While this ideal has not been practised by all young people at all times, evidence from the recent evaluation of the National HIV/AIDS Strategy in Australia (Feacham 1995) indicates that education programmes for youth appear to be working and that condom use is increasing. Surveys among university students in Sydney and Melbourne found that the percentage of 18- and 19-year-old students reporting that they always used condoms for vaginal sex with casual and regular partners increased between 1990 and 1994.

However, two large-scale surveys of different cohorts conducted in the United States documented an increase in sexual activity but no increase in condom use over the period 1988 to 1991 among young men (Ku et al. 1993) and a decrease in use from 1974 to 1991 among college-age men and women (Hale et al. 1993). Ku et al. concluded that early progress in fostering safer behaviours among young men slowed and possibly stopped in the 1990s, and recommended renewed prevention efforts. While the Australian data, at least, are encouraging, there is clearly no room for complacency about young people's sexual safety.

When we turn to individual change, the picture is not so promising. The findings from cross-sectional research have not been supported by the few longitudinal or follow-up studies that have measured change over time within the same individual (Kegeles et al. 1988; Rosenthal and Shepherd 1993). The studies have demonstrated that young people's resistance to messages about safe sex may be greater than is evidenced in cross-sectional studies. It would be inappropriate to place too much reliance on the few longitudinal studies that have been reported. Such studies are rare because of the high financial cost of such projects, the time involved in conducting them, and the potentially high drop-out rates. Furthermore, if the aim is to monitor change in sexual behaviours beginning with very young people, then the requirement to obtain parental consent may be problematic. Nevertheless, it is vital that these barriers be overcome so that research of this type is supported and carried out.

The progress of our education efforts should not be measured solely by their impact on behaviour. Central to the goal of promoting safe sexual practices is the need to ensure that attitudes and beliefs that underpin these practices are also modified. Indeed, without these changes, behaviour change is unlikely to occur. A climate where condoms are accepted as a routine means of disease prevention and where there is open discussion about, and acceptance of, sexual diversity is an essential prerequisite for creating a context for safe sex. It is already clear from research that putting HIV and AIDS on the educational agenda has increased young people's awareness of the need for sexual safety. Regardless of their actual use of condoms, many young people appear now to have discarded the old negative stereotypes of condoms as inhibiting good sex. These increasingly positive attitudes have not yet been translated into a less discriminatory view of those who are infected, and there is still a high level of stigma and shame attached to STDs of all types.

It is because education programmes have not been uniformly successful in all these areas that we have been forced to look beyond an individualistic perspective and towards identifying and addressing the critical social conditions that inhibit or facilitate sexual safety.

CHALLENGES FOR THE FUTURE

Will AIDS affect how you go about sex in the future?

Yes, I would pray that nothing ever happened. I think if a guy had AIDS, I think he would – I don't know – I don't think he would sleep with you if he knew he had AIDS. *(16-year-old female)*

While we still have young people expressing myths such as this, we cannot be complacent about our achievements.

Currently, standard HIV/AIDS education programmes draw heavily on Western middle-class values. But the assumptions behind these programmes may not fit the reality experienced by those most at risk. Research up to now has predominantly focused on convenience samples of high-school and university or college students. This has meant the exclusion from our knowledge base of the behaviours and beliefs of groups such as early school leavers, the unemployed, the homeless, intravenous drug users, and members of other minority groups. These young people are quite likely to be the most vulnerable to risk of infection. The sampling strategies used have also meant that young sexually active people below 16 years of age have been largely overlooked, as have those who are geographically isolated.

Young people are not part of one homogeneous group. We need to consider the broader societal factors that impact on youths' ability to accept and respond to safe-sex messages – factors such as poverty, culture, normative relationships between the sexes, and social alienation. For example, the fragile life circumstances of homeless teenagers – their lack of support, food, shelter and opportunities for intimate relationships – will inevitably affect the priority given to safe sex. An offer for food and shelter in exchange for unsafe sex may well be a powerful inducement, overriding long-term concerns about sexual health.

It has been said that HIV (and to some extent other STDs as well) constitutes many epidemics, not one. Seen within this context, the methods of approach must also be many and varied. For example, the solutions for reducing the spread of AIDS among young sex workers will involve different social interventions from those that assist young gay males to embrace self-acceptance and the corresponding self-esteem to choose safe-sex options. Breaking the nexus between adolescent girls' desires for romance and a perceived conflict over planning for sex requires a different approach from improving the housing and security of homeless young people so they do not feel pressured into selling sex. Encouraging responsible sexual options in cultures where women have little say in the matter is not a simple matter of public education about condoms, but must incorporate attention to the whole question of human rights.

The future development of education to prevent sexually transmitted diseases, including HIV, needs to take account of these issues. We would suggest, further, that the emphasis on disease, fear, shame and other negative constructions of sexuality have been counterproductive in gaining the commitment of young people to the safe-sex enterprise. We have not yet managed to describe the sexual culture in ways that effectively reflect or validate young people's lived experience. Their feelings of desire and longing can and often do create powerful anxieties for parents and other adults. It is not surprising, therefore, that these positive aspects of young people's developing sexuality are given little or no role in educational messages. If we can shift the emphasis from disease to sexual health, we can use fun, pleasure and intimacy, as well as responsibility, in the service of safe sex.

References

Abbott, S. (1987) *Talking About AIDS: A Report on the Issues of AIDS with Young Women*, Canberra: AIDS Action Council.
—— (1988) 'AIDS and young women', *The Bulletin of the National Clearinghouse for Youth Studies* 7: 38–41.
Abraham, C., Sheeran, P., Abrams, D., Spears, R., and Marks, D. (1991) 'Young people learning about AIDS: a study of beliefs and information sources', *Health Education Research* 6: 19–29.
Abrams, D., Abraham, C., Spears, R., and Marks, D. (1990) 'AIDS invulnerability, relationships, sexual behaviour and attitudes among 16 to 19 year olds', in P. Aggleton, P. Davies, and G. Hart (eds) *AIDS: Individual, Cultural and Policy Dimensions*, Lewes: Falmer Press.
Adelman, M.B. (1992) 'Sustaining passion: eroticism and safe-sex talk', *Archives of Sexual Behavior* 21: 481–94.
Adimara, A.A., Hamilton, H., Holmes, K.K., and Sparling, P.F. (1994) *Sexually Transmitted Diseases: Companion Handbook*, 2nd edn, New York: McGraw Hill.
Adler, N., Kegeles, S.M., and Genevro, J.L. (1992) 'Risk-taking and health', in J.F. Yates (ed.) *Risk-Taking Behavior*, New York: Wiley.
Ajzen, I., and Fishbein, M. (1977) 'Attitude–behaviour relations: a theoretical analysis and review of empirical research', *Psychological Bulletin* 84: 888–919.
—— (1980) *Understanding Attitudes and Predicting Social Behavior*, Englewood Cliffs, NJ: Prentice Hall.
Ajzen, I., and Madden, T.J. (1986) 'Prediction of goal directed behaviour: attitudes, intentions and perceived behaviour control', *Journal of Experimental and Social Psychology* 22: 453–74.
Altman, D. (1992a) 'AIDS and discourses of sexuality' in R.W. Connell and G.W. Dowsett (eds) *Rethinking Sex: Social Theory and Sexuality Research*, Melbourne: Melbourne University Press.
—— (1992b) 'The most political of diseases', in E. Timewell, V. Mininchiello, and D. Plummer (eds) *AIDS in Australia*, Sydney: Prentice Hall.
Anderson, M.D., and Christenson, G.M. (1991) 'Ethnic breakdown of AIDS-related knowledge and attitudes from the National Adolescent Student Health Survey', *Journal of Health Education* 22: 30–4.
Andre, T., and Bormann, L. (1991) 'Knowledge of Acquired Immunodefi-

150   Youth, AIDS, and STDs

ciency Syndrome and sexual responsibility among high school students', *Youth and Society* 22: 339–61.

Andrucci, G.L., Archer, R.P., Pancoast, D.L., and Gordon, R.A. (1989) 'The relationship of MMPI and Sensation Seeking Scales to adolescent drug use', *Journal of Personality Assessment* 53: 253–66.

Aneshensel, C.S., Fiedler, E.P., and Becarra, R.M. (1989) 'Fertility and fertility-related behavior among Mexican-American and non-Hispanic white female adolescents', *Journal of Health and Social Behavior* 30: 56–76.

Aral, S.O., and Holmes, K.K. (1990) 'Epidemiology of sexual behaviour and sexually transmitted diseases', in K.K. Holmes, P-A. Mardh, P.F. Sparling, P.J. Wiesner, W. Cates, S.M. Lemon, and W.E. Stamm (eds) *Sexually Transmitted Disease*, 2nd edn, New York: McGraw Hill.

Australian Broadcasting Commission (1993) *Report on Attitudes of Youth*, Canberra: Australian Broadcasting Commission.

Australian Doctor Weekly (1991) 'Teenage suicides doubled', *Australian Doctor Weekly* May 3.

Australian Institute of Family Studies (1981–2) *Australian Family Formation Project, Study 1: A Longitudinal Survey of Australians aged 13 to 34 years*, Canberra: Australian National University Social Science Data Archives.

Baldo, M., Aggeleton, P., and Slutkin, G. (1993) *Sex Education Does Not Lead to Earlier or Increased Sexual Activity in Youth*, Report to the World Health Organization Global Programme on AIDS, Geneva, Switzerland.

Bamford, E.J. (1935) *The House Not Made With Hands*, Melbourne.

Bandura, A. (1982) 'Self-efficacy mechanism in human agency', *American Psychologist* 37: 122–47.

Bartlett, J.G., and Finkbeiner, A.K. (1991) *The Guide to Living with HIV Infection*, Baltimore: Johns Hopkins University Press.

Bauman, K., and Udry, J.R. (1981) 'Subjective expected utility and adolescent sexual behavior', *Adolescence* 14: 527–38.

Becker, M.H. (1974) 'The health belief model and personal health behavior', *Health Education Monographs* 2: 326–473.

Becker, M.H., and Joseph, J.G. (1988) 'AIDS and behavioural change to reduce risk: a review', *American Journal of Public Health* 78: 394–410.

Bell, D., Feraios, A., and Bryan, T. (1990) 'Adolescent males' knowledge and attitudes about AIDS in the context of their social worlds', *Journal of Applied Social Psychology* 20: 424–48.

Benton, J.M., Mintzes, J.J., Kendrick, A.F., and Solomon, R.D. (1993) 'Alternative conceptions in sexually transmitted diseases: a cross-age study', *Journal of Sex Education and Therapy* 19: 165–82.

Blaney, N.T., Millon, C., Morgan, R., Eisdorfer, C., and Szapocznik, J. (1990) 'Emotional distress, stress-related disruption and coping among healthy HIV-positive gay males', *Psychology and Health* 4: 259–73.

Boldero, J.M., Moore, S.M., and Rosenthal, D.A. (1992) 'Intention, context, and safe sex: Australian adolescents' response to AIDS', *Journal of Applied Social Psychology* 22: 1357–97.

Bowler, S., Sheon, A.R., D'Angelo, L.J., and Vermund, S.H. (1992) 'HIV and AIDS risk among adolescents in the United States: increasing risk in the 90s', *Journal of Adolescence* 15: 345–71.

Boyer, C.B., and Kegeles, S.M. (1991) 'AIDS risk and prevention among adolescents', *Social Science and Medicine* 33: 11–23.

Brady, M., Baker, C., and Neinstein, L.S. (1988) 'Asymptomatic *Chalamydia trachomatis* infections in teenage males', *Journal of Adolescent Health Care* 9: 72–5.

Breakwell, G.M., and Fife-Schaw, C. (1991) 'Heterosexual anal intercourse and the risk of AIDS and HIV for 16–20-year-olds', *Health Education Journal* 50: 166–9.

—— (1992) 'Sexual activities and preferences in a United Kingdom sample of 16–20 year olds', *Archives of Sexual Behaviour* 21: 271–93.

—— (1994) 'Commitment to "safer" sex as a predictor of condom use among 16–20-year-olds', *Journal of Applied Social Psychology* 24: 189–217.

Brookman, R.R. (1990) 'Adolescent sexual behaviour', in K.K. Holmes, P-A. Mardh, P.F. Sparling, P.J. Wiesner, W. Cates, S.M. Lemon, and W.E. Stamm (eds) *Sexually Transmitted Disease*, 2nd edn, New York: McGraw Hill.

Brooks-Gunn, J., and Furstenberg, F.F. Jr. (1989) 'Adolescent sexual behavior', *American Psychologist* 44: 249–57.

Buhrich, N., Cooper, D.A., and Freed, E. (1988) 'HIV infection associated with symptoms indistinguishable from functional psychosis', *British Journal of Psychiatry* 152: 649–53.

Bury, J.K. (1991) 'Teenage sexual behaviour and the impact of AIDS', *Health Education Journal* 50: 43–9.

—— (1992) 'Pregnancy, heterosexual transmission, and contraception', in J. Bury, V. Morrison, and S. McLachlan (eds) *Working with Women and AIDS*, London: Routledge.

Buzwell, S. (1993) 'Unemployed young people's constructions of sexuality', unpublished report, Centre for the Study of Sexually Transmissible Diseases, La Trobe University, Melbourne, Australia.

Buzwell, S., Rosenthal, D.A., and Moore, S.M. (1992) 'Idealising the sexual experience', *Youth Studies Australia – HIV/AIDS Education* 1: 3–10.

Carmichael, I. (1995) 'Rights, duties and obligations in sex education', unpublished position paper, Baptist Churches of Tasmania, Tasmania, Australia.

Cass, V.C. (1979) 'Homosexual identity formation: a theoretical model', *Journal of Homosexuality* 4: 219–35.

Catania, J.A., Kegeles, S.M., and Coates, T.J. (1990) 'Towards an understanding of risk behavior: an AIDS risk reduction model (ARRM)' *Health Education Quarterly* 17: 53–72.

Cates, W. (1991) 'Teenagers and sexual risk-taking: the best of times and the worst of times', *Journal of Adolescent Health* 12: 84–94.

Centre for Adolescent Health (1992) *Adolescent Health Survey, 1992*, Melbourne: Centre for Adolescent Health, Melbourne University.

Chapman, S., and Hodgson, J. (1988) 'Showers in raincoats: attitudinal barriers to condom use in high risk heterosexuals', *Community Health Studies* 12: 97–105.

Chassin, L., Presson, C.C., and Sherman, S. (1989) 'Constructive vs destructive deviance in adolescent health-related behaviors', *Journal of Youth and Adolescence* 18: 245–62.

Chilman, C.S. (1980) *Adolescent Sexuality in a Changing American Society*, Maryland: US Department of Health, Education, and Welfare.

Cline, R., Johnson, S., and Freeman, K. (1992) 'Talk among sexual partners about AIDS: interpersonal communication for risk reduction or risk enhancement?', *Health Communication* 4: 39–56.

Cochran, S.D., and Mays, V.M. (1990) 'Sex, lies, and HIV', letter to the editor, *New England Journal of Medicine* 322: 774–5.

Coleman, J.C., and Hendry, L. (1990) *The Nature of Adolescence*, 2nd edn, London: Routledge.

Coles, P. (1989) 'French haemophiliacs awarded damages', *Nature* 340: 253.

Coles, R., and Stokes, G. (1985) *Sex and the American Teenager*, New York: Harper & Row.

Commonwealth Department of Community Services and Health (1986) *Australia's Response to AIDS*, Canberra: Commonwealth Department of Community Services and Health.

—— (1988) *National AIDS Education Campaign, Benchmark Survey 1986–1987 Summary Report 1: General Population and Adolescents*, Canberra: Commonwealth Department of Community Services and Health.

—— (1989) *National HIV/AIDS Strategy: A Policy Information Paper*, Canberra: Commonwealth Department of Community Services and Health.

—— (1992) *Report of the Evaluation of the National HIV/AIDS Strategy*, Canberra: Commonwealth Department of Community Services and Health.

Commonwealth Department of Health, Housing and Community Services (1992) *National Counselling Guidelines for HIV/AIDS*, Canberra: Commonwealth Department of Health, Housing and Community Services.

Congress of the United States, Office of Technological Assessment (1991) *Adolescent Health, Volume I: Summary and Policy Options*, Washington DC: Congress of the United States, Office of Technological Assessment.

Connell, R.W., and Kippax, S. (1990) 'Sexuality and the AIDS crisis: patterns of pleasure and practice in an Australian sample of gay and bisexual men', *The Journal of Sex Research* 27: 167–98.

Corey, L. (1990) 'Genital herpes', in K.K. Holmes, P-A. Mardh, P.F. Sparling, P.J. Wiesner, W. Cates, S.M. Lemon, and W.E. Stamm (eds) *Sexually Transmitted Disease*, 2nd edn, New York: McGraw Hill.

Crawford, J., Kippax, S., and Rodden, P. (1994) 'Knowledge and safe sex practice among heterosexual tertiary students as an outcome of socio-cultural change', paper given at the 10th International AIDS Conference, Yokohama, Japan, August.

Crawford, J., Turtle, A.M., and Kippax, S. (1990) 'Student favoured strategies for AIDS prevention', *Australian Journal of Psychology* 42: 123–38.

Dank, B.M. (1971) 'Coming out in the gay world', *Psychiatry* 34: 180–97.

Darling, C.A., and Hicks, M.W. (1982) 'Parental influence on adolescent sexuality: implications for parents as educators', *Journal of Youth and Adolescence* 11: 231–45.

David, H.P. (1993) 'European perspectives', paper given at the CPR/NICDH Workshop on Negotiating the Paths for Parenthood, Transnational Family Research Institute, Bethesda, MD, November.

Dean, L., Hall, W.E., and Martin, J.L. (1988) 'Chronic and intermittent AIDS-related bereavement in a panel of homosexual men in New York City', *Journal of Palliative Care* 4: 54–7.

de Graaf, R., Vanwesenbeeck, I., van Zessen, G., Straver, C.J., and Visser, J.H.

(1992) 'The effectiveness of condom use in heterosexual prostitution in The Netherlands', *AIDS* 7: 265–9.

Derelega, V.J., and Chaikin, A. (1975) *Sharing Intimacy: What We Reveal to Others and Why,* Englewood Cliffs, NJ: Prentice Hall.

Des Jarlais, D.C., Freidman, S.R., and Hopkins,W. (1985) 'Risk reduction for the acquired immunodeficiency syndrome amongst intravenous drug users', *Annals of Internal Medicine* 103: 755–9.

Devaney, B.L., and Hubley, K.S. (1981) *The Determinants of Adolescent Pregnancy and Childbearing,* Final report to the National Institute of Child Health and Human Development, Washington, DC.

Dew, M.A., Ragni, M.V., and Nimorwicz, P. (1990) 'Infection with human immunodeficiency virus and vulnerability to psychiatric distress: a study of men with hemophilia', *Archives of General Psychiatry* 47: 737–44.

DiClemente, R.J. (1992) 'Epidemiology of AIDS, HIV prevalence and HIV incidence among adolescents', *Journal of School Health* 62: 325–30.

—— (1993a) 'Psychosocial determinants of condom use among adolescents', in R.J. DiClemente (ed.) *Adolescents and AIDS: A Generation in Jeopardy,* Newbury Park, Calif.: Sage.

—— (1993b) *Adolescents and AIDS: A Generation in Jeopardy,* Newbury Park, Calif.: Sage.

DiClemente, R.J., Boyer, C.B., and Morales, E.S. (1988) 'Minorities and AIDS: knowledge, attitudes and misconceptions among Black and Latino adolescents', *American Journal of Public Health* 78: 55–7.

DiClemente, R.J., Zorn, J., and Temoshok, L. (1986) 'Adolescents and AIDS: a survey of knowledge, attitudes and beliefs about AIDS in San Francisco', *American Journal of Public Health* 76: 1443–5.

DiClemente, R.J., Lanier, M.M., Horan, P.F., and Lodico, M. (1991) 'Comparison of AIDS knowledge, attitudes, and behaviours among incarcerated adolescents and a public school sample in San Francisco', *American Journal of Public Health* 81: 628–30.

Donald, M., Lucke, J., Dunne, M., O'Toole, B., and Raphael, B. (1994) 'Determinants of condom use by Australian secondary students', *Journal of Adolescent Health* 15: 503–10.

Dryfoos, J. (1985) 'What the United States can learn about prevention of teenage pregnancy from other developed countries', *SIEC – US Report* 14(2): 1–7.

—— (1990) *Adolescents at Risk: Prevalence and Prevention,* New York: Oxford University Press.

Dunne, M., Donald, M., Lucke, J., Nilsson, R., and Raphael, B. (1993a) *National HIV/AIDS Evaluation 1992 HIV Risk and Sexual Behaviour Survey in Australian Secondary Schools: Final Report,* Canberra: Commonwealth Department of Health and Community Services.

Dunne, M., Donald, M., Lucke, J., and Raphael, B. (1993b) 'The sexual behaviour of young people in rural Australia', in K. Malko (ed.) *A Fair Go for Rural Health – Forward Together: 2nd National Rural Health Conference,* Canberra: Australian Government Publishing Service.

Dusek, J.B. (1991) *Adolescent Development and Behavior,* Englewood Cliffs, NJ: Prentice Hall.

Ehrhardt, A.A. (1993) 'Sex education for young people', *National AIDS Bulletin* 7(6): 32–5.

154   Youth, AIDS, and STDs

Ehrhardt, A.A., and Wasserheit, J.N. (1992) 'Age, gender and sexual risk behaviours for sexually transmitted diseases in the United States', in J.N. Wasserheit, S.O. Aral, and K.K. Holmes (eds) *Research Issues in Human Behaviour and Sexually Transmitted Diseases in the AIDS Era*, Washington, DC: American Society of Microbiology.

Elkind, D. (1967) 'Egocentrism in adolescence', *Child Development* 38: 1025–34.

Ellickson, P.L., Lara, M.E., Sherbourne, C.D., and Zima, B. (1993) *Forgotten Ages, Forgotten Problems*, Santa Monica, Calif.: Rand.

Erikson, E. (1959) 'Identity and the life cycle', *Psychological Issues* 1: 1–71.

—— (1968) *Identity, Youth and Crisis*, New York: Norton.

Fahey, J., and Mitchell, A. (1995) 'The contribution of talkback radio sex shows to the construction of the sexual world and sexual health of adolescent listeners', manuscript under review.

Farmer, P. (1992) *AIDS and Accusation: Haiti and the Geography of Blame*, Los Angeles: University of California Press.

Faulstich, M.E. (1987) 'Psychiatric aspects of AIDS', *American Journal of Psychiatry* 144: 551–6

Feacham, R.G.A. (1995) *Valuing the Past ... Investing in the Future: Evaluation of the National HIV/AIDS Strategy 1993–94 to 1995–96*, Canberra: Commonwealth Department of Human Services and Health.

Feldman, S.S., and Brown, N. (1993) 'Family influence on adolescent male sexuality: the mediational role of self-restraint', *Social Development* 2: 15–35.

Feldman, S.S., and Elliott, G. (1990) *At the Threshold: The Developing Adolescent*, Cambridge, Mass.: Harvard University Press.

Fennell, R. (1993) 'A review of evaluations of peer education programs', *Journal of American College Health* 41: 251–3.

Ferrara, A.J. (1984) 'My personal experience with AIDS', *American Psychologist* 39: 1285–7.

Fine, M. (1988) 'Sexuality, schooling, and adolescent females: the missing discourse of desire', *Harvard Educational Review* 58: 29–53.

Forrest, D.J., and Silverman, J. (1989) 'When public school teachers teach about preventing pregnancy, AIDS and sexually transmitted diseases', *Family Planning Perspectives* 21: 65–72.

Foucault, M. (1973) *The Birth of the Clinic*, trans. A. Sheridan, New York: Pantheon.

Frankham, J., and Stronach, I. (1990) *Making a Drama Out of a Crisis: An Evaluation of the Norfolk Action Against Aids Health Education Play 'Love Bites'*, Norwich: Centre for Applied Research in Education, University of East Anglia.

Fullilove, R.E., Fullilove, M.T., and Bowser, B.P. (1990) 'Risk of sexually transmitted disease among black adolescent crack users in Oakland and San Francisco, California', *Journal of the American Medical Association* 263: 851–5.

Galligan, R., and Terry, D. (1993) 'Romantic ideals, fear of negative implications, and the practice of safe sex', *Journal of Applied Social Psychology* 23: 1685–1711.

Gallois, C., Kashima, Y., Hills, R., and McCamish, M. (1990) 'Preferred strategies for safe sex: relation to past and actual behaviour among sexually active men and women', paper given at the Sixth International Conference on AIDS, San Francisco, June.

References 155

Gallois, C., Kashima, Y., Terry, D., McCamish, M., Timmins, P., and Chauvin, A. (1992a) 'Safe and unsafe sexual intentions and behaviour: the effects of norms and attitudes', *Journal of Applied Social Psychology* 22: 1521–45.

Gallois, C., Statham, D., and Smith, S. (1992b) *Women and HIV/AIDS Education in Australia*, Canberra: Commonwealth Department of Health and Human Services.

Garland, S.M., Gertig, M., and McInnes, J.A. (1993) 'Genital *chlamydia trachomatis* infection in Australia', *The Medical Journal of Australia* 159: 90–6.

Gerety, R.J., and Barker, L.F. (1976) 'Viral antigens and antibodies in hemophiliacs', in *National Heart, Lung, and Blood Institute: Unsolved Therapeutic Problems in Hemophilia*, Washington, DC: U.S. Government Printing Office.

Geringer, W.M., Marks, S., Allen, W.J., and Armstrong, K.A. (1993) 'Knowledge, attitudes and behaviours related to condom use and STDs in a high risk population', *Journal of Sex Research* 30: 75–83.

Gilbert, P., and Taylor, S. (1991) *Fashioning the Feminine: Girls, Popular Culture and Schooling*, Sydney: Allen & Unwin.

Glaun, D. (1991) 'Development of CF and the healthy children's concepts of illness and the body', unpublished thesis, Department of Psychology, University of Melbourne, Melbourne, Australia.

Goggin, M. (1989) 'Intimacy, sexuality, and sexual behaviour among young Australian adults', unpublished thesis, Department of Psychology, University of Melbourne, Melbourne, Australia.

—— (1993) 'Gay and lesbian adolescence', in S.M. Moore and D.A. Rosenthal *Sexuality in Adolescence*, London: Routledge.

Gold, R. (1993) 'On the need to mind the gap: on-line versus off-line cognitions underlying sexual risk-taking', in D.J. Terry, C. Gallois, and M. McCamish (eds) *The Theory of Reasoned Action: Its Application to AIDS Preventive Behaviour*, Oxford: Pergamon Press.

Gold, R.S., Skinner, M.J., Grant, P.J., and Plummer, D.C. (1991) 'Situational factors and thought processes associated with unprotected intercourse in gay men', *Psychology and Health* 5: 259–78.

Goldman, R.J., and Goldman, J.D.G. (1988) *Show Me Yours: Understanding Children's Sexuality*, Ringwood: Penguin.

Grant, D., and Anns, M. (1988) 'Counseling AIDS antibody positive clients: reactions and treatment', *American Psychologist* 43: 72–4.

Greig, R., and Raphael, B. (1989) 'AIDS prevention and adolescents', *Community Health Studies* 13: 211–7.

Grimes, D.A. (1986) 'Deaths due to sexually transmitted diseases', *Journal of the American Medical Association* 255: 1727–9.

Gunn, D., and Guyomard, P. (eds) (1990) *A Young Girl's Diary: A New Edition*, London: Unwin Hyman.

Gurien, R. (1994) 'Conversations about their safe sex behaviors', paper given at the Conference of Language and Social Psychology, Brisbane, Australia, July.

Hadley, S. (1994) 'Tertiary student drinking patterns: prediction of risky drinking behaviour in a university setting', unpublished MEd Studies thesis, Monash University, Melbourne, Australia.

Haffner, D. (1992) 'Youth still at risk, yet barriers to education remain: SIECUS

156   Youth, AIDS, and STDs

testimony for the National AIDS Commission', *SIECUS Report* November/December.

Hale, R.W., Char, D.F., Nagy, K., and Stockert, N. (1993) 'Seventeen-year review of sexual and contraceptive behavior on a college campus', *American Journal of Obstetrics and Gynaecology* 168: 1833–8.

Harris, M.B., Harris, R.J., and Davis, S.M. (1991) 'Ethnic and gender differences in southwestern students' sources of information about health', *Health Education Research* 6: 31–42.

Hart, G. (1993) 'STD epidemiology in Australasia: the old and the new', *Venereology* 6: 5–9.

Henry, S. (1995) 'No sex please, we're teenagers', *Good Weekend: The Age Magazine*, May 13: 42–6.

Herek, G.M. (1984) 'Beyond "homophobia": a social psychological perspective on attitudes towards lesbians and gay men', *Journal of Homosexuality* 10: 1–21.

Herek, G.M., and Glunt, E.K. (1995) 'An epidemic of stigma: public reaction to AIDS', in E.R. Bethel (ed.) *AIDS: Readings on a Global Crisis*, Boston: Allyn & Bacon.

Hersch, P. (1988) 'Coming of age on city streets', *Psychology Today* 22: 28–37.

Hingson, R., and Strunin, L. (1992) 'Monitoring adolescents' responses to the AIDS epidemic: changes in knowledge, attitudes, beliefs, and behaviours', in R.J. DiClemente (ed.) *Adolescents and Aids: A Generation in Jeopardy*, Newbury Park, Calif.: Sage.

Hingson, R., Strunin, L., Berlin, B., and Heerin, T. (1990) 'Beliefs about AIDS, use of alcohol and drugs, and unprotected sex among Massachusetts adolescents', *American Journal of Public Health* 80: 295–9.

Hingson, R., Strunin, L., Grady, M., Strunk, N., Carr, R., Berlin, B., and Craven, D.E. (1991) 'Knowledge about HIV and behavioural risks of foreign-born Boston public school students', *American Journal of Public Health* 81: 1638–41.

Hofferth, S.L., and Hayes, C.D. (eds) (1987) *Risking the Future: Adolescent Sexuality, Pregnancy and Childbearing* 1, Washington, DC: National Academy of Science.

Hofferth, S.L., Kahn, J., and Baldwin, W. (1987) 'Premarital sexual activity among U.S. teenage women', *Family Planning Perspectives* 19: 46–53.

Holland, J., Ramazanoglu, C., Scott, S., Sharpe, S., and Thomson, R. (1990a) '*Don't Die of Ignorance – I Nearly Died of Embarrassment' Condoms in Context*, The Womens Risk AIDS Project, paper no. 2. London: Tufnell Press.

—— (1990b) 'Sex, gender and power: young women's sexuality in the shadow of AIDS', *Sociology of Health and Illness* 12: 336–50.

Holland, J.C., Jacobsen, P., and Breitbart, W. (1992) 'Psychiatric and psychosocial aspects of HIV infection', in V.T. Devita, Jr., S. Hellman, and S.A. Rosenberg (eds) *AIDS: Etiology, Diagnosis, Treatment and Prevention*, Philadelphia: J.B. Lippincott.

Holmes, K.K., Mardh, P-A., Sparling, P.F., Wiesner, P.J., Cates, W., Lemon, S.M., and Stamm, W.E. (eds) (1990) *Sexually Transmitted Disease*, 2nd edn, New York: McGraw Hill.

Howard, J. (1991) 'Dulling the pain: two surveys of Sydney street youth', paper given at the Ninth National Behavioural Medicine Conference on Adolescence and Health, Sydney, Australia, October.

Ingham, R., Woodcock, A., and Stenner, K. (1991) 'Getting to know you ...
young people's knowledge of their partners at first intercourse', *Journal of
Community and Applied Psychology* 1: 117–32.

Irwin, C.E., Jr. (1993) 'Adolescence and risk taking: how are they related', in
N.J. Bell and R.W. Bell (eds.) *Adolescent Risk Taking*, Newbury Park, Calif.:
Sage.

Irwin, C.E., Jr., and Millstein, S.G. (1986) 'Biopsychosocial correlates of risk-
taking behaviors during adolescence', *Journal of Adolescent Health Care* 7:
82–96.

Jaccard, J., and Davidson, A.R. (1972) 'Toward an understanding of family
planning behaviors: an initial investigation', *Journal of Applied Social
Psychology* 2: 228–35.

Janz, N.K., and Becker, M.H. (1984) 'The Health Belief Model a decade later',
Health Education Quarterly 11: 1–47.

Jessor, S.L., and Jessor, R. (1977) *Problem Behavior and Psychosocial Development:
A Longitudinal Study of Youth*, New York: Academic Press.

Johnson, A.M., Wadsworth, J., Wellings, K., and Field, J. (1994) *Sexual
Attitudes and Lifestyles*, Oxford: Blackwell Scientific.

Jones, R.B., and Wasserheit, J.N. (1991) 'Introduction to the biology and
natural history of sexually transmitted diseases', in J.N. Wasserheit, S.O.
Aral, and K.K. Holmes (eds) *Research Issues in Human Behavior and Sexually
Transmitted Diseases in the AIDS Era*, Washington, DC: American Society for
Microbiology.

Kashima, Y., Gallois, C., and McCamish, M. (1992) 'Predicting the use of
condoms: past behavior, norms and the sexual partner', in T. Edgar, M.A.
Fitzpatrick, and V.S. Freimuth (eds) *AIDS: A Communication Perspective*,
Hillsdale, NJ: Lawrence Erlbaum Associates.

Katz, S. (1995) 'HIV testing – a phony cure', in E.R. Bethel (ed.) *AIDS: Readings
on a Global Crisis*, Boston: Allyn & Bacon.

Kegeles, S., Adler, N., and Irwin, C. (1988) 'Sexually active adolescents and
condoms: knowledge, attitudes and changes over one year', *American
Journal of Public Health* 78: 260–1.

Keller, S.E., Schleifer, S.J., Bartlett, J.A., and Johnson, R.L. (1988) 'The sexual
behaviour of adolescents and risk of AIDS', *Journal of the American Medical
Association* 260: 5386.

Kent, V., Davies, M., Deverall, K., and Gottesman, S. (1990) 'Social interaction
routines involved in heterosexual encounters: prelude to first intercourse',
paper given at 4th Conference on Social Aspects of AIDS, London, April.

King, A., Beazley, R., Warren, W., Hankins, C., Robertson, A., and Radford, J.
(1989) 'Highlights from the Canada youth and AIDS study', *Journal of
School and Health* 59: 139–45.

Kinsey, A.C., Pomeroy, W.B., and Martin, C.E. (1948) *Sexual Behavior in the
Human Male*, Philadelphia: Saunders.

Kinsey, A.C., Pomeroy, W.B., Martin, C.E., and Gebhard, P.H. (1953) *Sexual
Behavior in the Human Female*, Philadelphia: Saunders.

Kippax, S., Crawford, J., and Walby, C. (1994) 'Heterosexuality, masculinity
and HIV: barriers to safe heterosexual practice', *AIDS* 8 (Supp. 1): 315.

Kirby, D. (1992) 'School-based prevention programs: design, evaluation, and
effectiveness' in R.J. DiClemente (ed.) *Adolescents and AIDS: A Generation in
Jeopardy*, Newbury Park, Calif.: Sage.

158   Youth, AIDS, and STDs

Kirby, D., Short, L., Collins, J., Rugg, D., Kolbe, L., Howard, M., Miller, B., Sonenstein, F., and Zabin, L. (1994) 'School-based programs to reduce sexual risk behaviours: a review of effectiveness', *Public Health Reports* 109: 339–60.

Klee, H. (1990) 'Some observations on the sexual behaviour of injecting drug users: implications for the spread of HIV infection', in P. Aggleton, P. Davies, and G. Hart (eds) *AIDS: Individual, Cultural and Policy Dimensions*, Lewes: Falmer Press.

Klitsch, M. (1990) 'Teenagers' condom use affected by peer factors, not health concerns', *Family Planning Perspectives* 22: 95.

Kovacs, G.T., Westcott, M., Rusden, J., Asche, V., King, H., Haynes, S.E., Moore, E.K., and Ketelbey, J.W. (1987) 'The prevalence of *chlamydia trachomatis* in a young sexually active population', *The Medical Journal of Australia* 147: 550–2.

Ku, L., Sonenstein, F.L., and Pleck, J.H. (1993) 'Young men's risk behaviors for HIV infection and sexually transmitted diseases, 1988 through 1991', *American Journal of Public Health* 83: 1609–15.

Kubler-Ross, E. (1970) *On Death and Dying*, London: Tavistock.

—— (1987) *AIDS – The Ultimate Challenge*, New York: Macmillan.

Leap, N., and Hunter, B. (1993) *The Midwife's Tale*, London: Scarlet Press.

Lee, C. (1983) *The Ostrich Position: Sex, Schooling and Mystification*, London: Writers and Readers Publishing Co-operative.

Lemon, S.M., and Newbold, J.E. (1990) 'Viral hepatitis', in K.K. Holmes, P.-A. Mardh, P.F. Sparling, P.J. Wiesner, W. Cates, S.M. Lemon, and W.E. Stamm (eds) *Sexually Transmitted Disease*, 2nd edn, New York: McGraw Hill.

Lenehan, Lynton, Bloom, and Blaxland (Market Research) (1992) *Exploring What Youth Understands 'Safe Sex' and 'Safer Sex' to Mean*, Report to Department of Health, Housing and Community Services, Sydney, Australia.

Levenson, M.R. (1990) 'Risk-taking and personality', *Journal of Personality and Social Psychology* 58: 1073–80.

Levitt, M.Z., Selman, R.L., and Richmond, J.B. (1991) 'The psychosocial foundations of early adolescents' high-risk behavior: implications for research and practice', *Journal of Research on Adolescence* 1: 349–78.

Lhuede, D., and Moore, S.M. (1994) 'AIDS vulnerability of homeless youth', *Venereology* 7: 117–23.

Louie, R., Rosenthal, D.A., and Crofts, N. (1996) 'Injecting and sexual risk-taking among young injecting drug users', *Venereology*, in press.

Loxley, W., and Ovenden, P. (1992) '"I wouldn't share": teenage injecting drug users in Perth and HIV/AIDS prevention', paper given at the 3rd International Conference on the Reduction of Drug Related Harm, Perth, April.

Lucke, J., Dunne, M., Donald, M., and Raphael, B. (1993) 'Knowledge of STDs and perceived risk of infection: a study of Australian youth', *Venereology* 6: 57–63.

MacCallum, L.R., France, A.J., Jones, M.E., Steel, C.M., Burns, S.M., and Brettle, R.P. (1988) 'The effects of pregnancy on the progression of HIV infection', paper given at IVth International Conference on AIDS, Stockholm, June.

McCamish, M. (1992) *Results of Student Survey on AIDS Knowledge and Beliefs at the University of Queensland*, Report to the University of Queensland Vice Chancellor's Committee AIDS Working Party, Brisbane, Australia.

McKeganey, N., and Barnard, M. (1990) 'Drug injectors' risks for HIV', in P. Aggleton, P. Davis, and G. Hart (eds) *AIDS: Individual, Cultural and Policy Dimensions*, Lewes: Falmer Press.

McKenzie, J., Goggin, M., and Rosemeyer, D. (1992) *When You Say Yes Report: Safe Sex Campaign Evaluation of the Victorian AIDS Council Youth Programme*, Melbourne: Victorian AIDS Council.

McLeod, J., and Nott, P. (1994) *A Place to Belong: Gay Community Attachment in Young Men Who Have Sex With Men, and the Prevention of HIV Infection*, Report to the Australian Federation of AIDS Organisations, Sydney, Australia.

McRobbie, A. (1991) *From 'Jackie' to 'Just Seventeen'*, London: Macmillan.

Masters, W., and Johnson, V. (1970) *Human Sexual Inadequacy*, London: Churchill.

Matthews, B.R., Richardson, K.D., Price, J., and Williams, G. (1990) 'Homeless youth and AIDS: knowledge, attitudes and behaviour', *The Medical Journal of Australia* 153: 20–3.

Mays, V.M., and Cochran, S.D. (1993) 'Ethnic and gender differences in beliefs about sex partner questioning to reduce HIV risk', *Journal of Adolescent Research* 8: 77–88.

Mertz, G.J., Coombs, R.W., Ashley, R., Jourden, J., Remington, M., Winter, C., Fahnlander, A., Guinan, M., Ducey, H., and Corey, L. (1988) 'Transmission of genital herpes in couples with one symptomatic and one asymptomatic partner: a prospective study', *Journal of Infectious Diseases* 157: 1169–77.

Metzler, C.W., Noell, J., and Biglan, A. (1992) 'The validation of a construct of high-risk sexual behavior in heterosexual adults', *Journal of Adolescent Research* 7: 233–49.

Mindel, A. (1995) 'Genital HPV infection: slow progress', *Venereology* 8: 164–5.

Minichiello, V., Paxton, S., Cowlings, V., Cross, G., Savage, J., Sculthorpe, A., and Cairns, B. (1994) 'Young people's knowledge of STDs: labels, transmission and symptoms', paper given at the Australasian Sexual Health Conference, Queensland, April.

Misson, R. (1994) 'Every newsstand has them: teaching popular teenage magazines', in B. Corcoran, M. Hayhoe, and G. Pradl (eds) *Knowledge in the Making: Challenging the Text in the Classroom*, Portsmouth, NH: Heinemann Boynton/Cook.

Mitchell, A., and Rosenthal, D.A. (1994) *Report of National Workshop on the HIV/AIDS Needs of Homeless Young People*, Report to Commonwealth Department of Human Services and Health, Canberra, Australia.

Moore, K., Peterson, J., and Furstenberg, F., Jr. (1986) 'Parental attitudes and the occurrence of early sexual activity', *Journal of Marriage and the Family* 48: 777–82.

Moore, S.M. (1994) 'Parents' contributions to girls' sexuality education', paper given at the 29th Annual Conference of the Australian Psychological Society, Wollongong, September.

Moore, S.M., and Barling, N. (1991) 'Developmental status and AIDS attitudes in adolescence', *Journal of Genetic Psychology* 152: 5–16.

Moore, S.M., and Gullone, E. (1995) 'Predicting adolescent risk behaviour

160   *Youth, AIDS, and STDs*

using a personalised cost–benefit analysis', *Journal of Youth and Adolescence,* in press.

Moore, S.M., and Rosenthal, D.A. (1991a) 'Adolescent invulnerability and perception of AIDS risk', *Journal of Adolescent Research* 6: 160–80.

—— (1991b) 'Adolescents' perceptions of friends' and parents' attitude to sex and sexual risk-taking', *Journal of Community and Applied Psychology* 1: 189–200.

—— (1991c) 'Condoms and coitus: adolescent attitudes to AIDS and safe sex behaviour', *Journal of Adolescence* 14: 211–27.

—— (1992a) 'Australian adolescents' perceptions of health related risks', *Journal of Adolescent Research* 7: 177–91.

—— (1992b) 'The social context of adolescent sexuality study', unpublished interviews.

—— (1993a) 'The social context of adolescent sexuality: safe sex implications', *Journal of Adolescence* 15: 415–35.

—— (1993b) 'Venturesomeness, impulsiveness, and risky behavior among older adolescents', *Perceptual and Motor Skills* 76: 98.

—— (1995a) 'Love, sex and passion among single heterosexuals', manuscript in preparation.

—— (1995b) 'Young people assess their risk of sexually transmissible diseases', *Psychology and Health,* in press.

Morris, R.E., Baker, C.J., and Huscroft, S. (1992) 'Incarcerated youth at risk for HIV infection', in R.J. DiClemente (ed.) *Adolescents and AIDS: A Generation in Jeopardy,* Newbury Park, Calif.: Sage.

Morrison, D. (1985) 'Adolescent contraceptive behaviour: a review', *Psychological Bulletin* 98: 538–68.

National Centre in HIV Epidemiology and Clinical Research (1994), *Australian HIV Surveillance Report* 10: 1–36.

National Health and Medical Research Council (1992) *Health Needs of Homeless Youth: A Summary of Key Issues for Those Developing Policies or Providing Services for Young Homeless People,* Canberra: National Health and Medical Research Council.

Neustatter, W.L. (1954) 'Homosexuality: the medical aspects', *Practitioner* 172: 364–73.

New South Wales Department of Health (1994) *Guidelines for the Conduct of Peer Education Programs,* Sydney: New South Wales Department of Health.

Newcomer, S.J., and Udry, J.R. (1983) 'Adolescent sexual behavior and popularity', *Adolescence* 18: 515–22.

—— (1985) 'Oral sex in an adolescent population', *Archives of Sexual Behavior* 14: 41–6.

O'Campo, P., Deboer, M., Faden, R.R., Kass, N., Gielen, A.C., and Anderson, J. (1992) 'Prior episode of sexually transmitted disease and subsequent risk-reduction interventions', *Sexually Transmitted Diseases* 19: 326–30.

O'Connell, J.K., Price, J.H., Roberts, S.M., Jurs, S.G., and McKinley, R. (1985) 'Utilising the Health Belief Model to predict dieting and exercising behavior of obese and non-obese adolescents', *Health Education Quarterly* 12: 343–51.

O'Donnell, M., and Jackson, A. (1990) *A Peer Education Approach to HIV/AIDS Prevention: An Evaluative Study,* Report to the Australian Federation of AIDS Organisations, Sydney, Australia.

O'Keefe, T., and Walker, I. (1992) *Being Positive: Living with HIV/AIDS*, Sydney: ABC Enterprises.

Ollis, D. (1995) *STD/AIDS Prevention Education Position Paper*, Melbourne: Victorian Directorate of School Education.

Omelczuk, S., Underwood, R., and White, R. (1991) 'Issues confronting youth in remote communities', paper given at the Australian Association for Adolescent Health Biennial Conference, Brisbane, May.

Oriel, D. (1990) 'Genital human papillomavirus infection', in K.K. Holmes, P-A. Mardh, P.F. Sparling, P.J. Wiesner, W. Cates, S.M. Lemon, and W.E. Stamm (eds) *Sexually Transmitted Disease*, 2nd edn, New York: McGraw Hill.

Orr, D.P., Langedeld, C.D., Katz, B.P., Caine, V.A., Dias, P., Blythe, M., and Jones, R.B. (1992) 'Factors associated with condom use among sexually active female adolescents', *Journal of Pediatrics* 120: 311–7.

Palmer, G., and Short, S. (1994) *Health Care and Public Policy: An Australian Analysis*, Melbourne: MacMillan.

Patton, W., and Mannison, M. (1995) 'Sexual coercion in dating situations among university students: preliminary Australian data', *Australian Journal of Psychology* 47: 66–72.

Peart, R., Rosenthal, D.A., and Mitchell, A. (1995) 'Pressure or pleasure? Young people negotiating a sexual encounter', manuscript under review.

Perry, S.W. (1990) 'Organic mental disorders caused by HIV: update on early diagnosis and treatment', *American Journal of Psychiatry* 147: 696–704.

Pleck, J.H., Sonenstein, F.L., and Ku, L.C. (1993) 'Masculine ideology: its impact on adolescent males' heterosexual relationships', *Journal of Social Issues* 49: 11–29.

Plummer, D., Kovacs, G., and Westmore, A. (1995) *Sexually Transmitted Diseases*, Melbourne: Hill of Content.

Porter, R., and Hall, L. (1995) *The Facts of Life: The Creation of Sexual Knowledge in Britain 1650–1950*, London: Yale University Press.

Potter, J., and Wetherall, M. (1987) *Discourse and Social Psychology: Beyond Attitudes and Behaviour*, London: Sage.

Pyett, P. (1995) *Living with Herpes: A Report to the Melbourne Herpes Self Help Group (HELM)*, Melbourne: Centre for the Study of Sexually Transmissible Diseases, La Trobe University.

Reiser, C. (1986) 'Herpes: a physical and moral dilemma', *College Student Journal* 20: 260–9.

Reulbach, W. (1991) 'Counseling chemically dependent HIV positive adolescents', *Journal of Chemical Dependency Treatment* 4: 31–43.

Richard, R., and van der Pligt, J. (1991) 'Factors affecting condom use among adolescents', *Journal of Community and Applied Social Psychology* 1: 105–16.

Richie, N., and Getty, A. (1994) 'Did an AIDS peer education program change first year college students' behaviour?', *Journal of American College Health* 42: 163–5.

Rickert, V.I., Jay, M.S., and Gottleib, A. (1991) 'Effects of a peer-counselled AIDS education program on knowledge, attitudes, and satisfaction of adolescents', *Journal of Adolescent Health* 12: 38–43.

Roberts, C., Kippax, S., Spongberg, M., and Crawford, J. (1996) '"Going down": oral sex, imaginary bodies and HIV', *AIDS and Culture*, in press.

162   *Youth, AIDS, and STDs*

Robinson, J. (ed.) (1993) *'Becoming Aware . . .': Women and HIV/AIDS*, Deakin, ACT: Family Planning Australia.

Robinson, R. (1994) *Safe Syringe Disposal – A Community Response: A Handbook for Victorian Local Government*, Melbourne: Centre for Social Health.

Rogel, J., Zuehlke, M.E., Peterson, A.C., Tobin-Richards, M., and Shelton, M. (1980) 'Contraceptive behavior in adolescence: a decision-making perspective', *Journal of Youth and Adolescence* 9: 491–506.

Rosenstock, I.M. (1974) 'The Health Belief Model and preventive health behavior', *Health Education Monographs* 2: 354–86.

Rosenthal, D.A., and Collis, F. (1996) 'Parents' beliefs about adolescent sexuality and HIV/AIDS', *Journal of HIV/AIDS Prevention and Education for Adolescents and Children*, in press.

Rosenthal, D.A., and Moore, S.M. (1991) 'Risky business: adolescents and HIV/AIDS', *The Bulletin for the National Clearinghouse of Youth Studies* 10: 20–5.

—— (1993) 'Myths and rationality: adolescents' decisions to have safe sex', paper given at the 9th International AIDS Conference, Berlin, June.

—— (1994) 'Stigma and ignorance: young people's beliefs about STDs', *Venereology* 7: 62–6.

—— (1995) 'The singles scene study', unpublished interviews.

Rosenthal, D.A., and Reichler, H. (1994) *Young Heterosexuals, HIV/AIDS, and STDs*, Canberra: Department of Human Services and Health.

Rosenthal, D.A., and Shepherd, H. (1993) 'A six month followup of Australian adolescents' sexual risk taking, HIV/AIDS knowledge, and attitudes to condoms', *Journal of Community and Applied Social Psychology* 3: 53–65.

Rosenthal, D.A., and Smith, A.M.A. (1994) 'Adolescents and sexually transmissible diseases: information sources, preferences and trust', manuscript under review.

Rosenthal, D.A., Moore, S.M., and Brumen, I. (1990) 'Ethnic group differences in adolescents' responses to AIDS', *Australian Journal of Social Issues* 25: 220–39.

Rosenthal, D.A., Moore, S.M., and Flynn, I. (1991) 'Adolescent self-efficacy, self-esteem and sexual risk taking', *Journal of Community and Applied Social Psychology* 1: 77–88.

Rosenthal, D.A., Hall, C., and Moore, S.M. (1992) 'AIDS, adolescents, and sexual risk taking: a test of the Health Belief Model', *Australian Psychologist* 27: 166–71.

Rosenthal, D.A., Moore, S.M., and Buzwell, S. (1994) 'Homeless youths: sexual and drug related behaviour, sexual beliefs and HIV/AIDS risk', *AIDS Care* 6: 83–94.

Rosenthal, D.A., Moore, S.M., and Fernbach, M. (1996a) 'The singles scene: safe sex practices and attitudes among at-risk heterosexual adults', *Psychology and Health*, in press.

Rosenthal, D.A., Smith, A.M.A., Reichler, H., and Moore, S.M. (1996b) 'Changes in young people's HIV-related knowledge, attitudes and behaviours, 1989–1994', *Genitourinary Medicine*, in press.

Rosenthal, D.A., Waters, L., and Glaun, D. (1996c) 'What do pre-adolescents understand about HIV/AIDS?', *Psychology and Health* 10: 507–22.

Rosenthal, D.A., Moore, S.M., and Gifford, S. (1996d) 'Safe sex or safe love? Incompatible opposites', manuscript under review.

Ross, M.W. (1990) 'Psychological determinants of increased condom use and safer sex in homosexual men: a longitudinal study', *International Journal of STDs and AIDS* 1: 98–101.

Ross, M.W., Tebble, W., and Viliunas, D. (1989) 'Staging of psychological reactions to HIV infection in asymptomatic homosexual men', *Journal of Psychology and Human Sexuality* 2: 93–104.

Rotheram-Borus, M.J., and Koopman, C. (1991) 'Sexual risk behaviours, AIDS knowledge, and beliefs about AIDS among runaways', *American Journal of Public Health* 81: 208–10.

Rotheram-Borus, M.J., Becker, J.V., Koopman, C., and Kaplan, M. (1991) 'AIDS knowledge and beliefs, and sexual behaviour of sexually delinquent and non-delinquent (runaway) adolescents', *Journal of Adolescence* 14: 229–44.

St Lawrence, J.S. (1993) 'African-American adolents' knowledge, health-related attitudes, sexual behaviour, and contraceptive decisions: implications for the prevention of adolescent HIV infection', *Journal of Consulting and Clinical Psychology* 61: 104–12.

Schmidt, G., Klusmann, D., Zeitzschel, U., and Lange, C. (1994) 'Changes in adolescents' sexuality between 1970 and 1990 in West Germany', *Archives of Sexual Behaviour* 23: 489–513.

Schoenbaum, E.E., Davenny, K., and Selwyn, P.A. (1988) 'The impact of pregnancy on HIV-related disease', in C. Hudson and F. Sharp (eds) *AIDS and Obstetrics and Gynaecology*, London: Royal College of Obstetricians and Gynaecologists.

Schofield, M. (1965) *The Sexual Behaviour of Young People*, London: Longmans.

Scott, A., and Griffin, H. (1989) *Concept Testing the Dundee 'Condoms in AIDS Prevention' Initiative*, Dundee: University of Strathclyde Advertising Research Unit.

Sears, J.T. (1992) 'Educators, homosexuality, and homosexual students: are personal feelings related to professional beliefs?', in K.M. Harbeck (ed.) *Coming Out of the Classroom Closet: Gay and Lesbian Students, Teachers and Curricula*, New York: The Harvard Press.

Short, R.V. (1993) 'The AIDS epidemic: what are the priorities?', paper given at the VIIIth World Congress on Human Reproduction, Bali, April.

Silbereisen, R.K., and Noack, P. (1988) 'On the constructive role of problem behaviour in adolescence/childhood', in N. Bolger, A. Caspi, G. Downey, and M. Moorehouse (eds) *Person and Context: Developmental Process*, Cambridge: Cambridge University Press.

Slap, B., Plotkin, S., Khalid, N., and Michelman, D. (1991) 'A human immunodefficiency virus peer education program for adolescent females', *Journal of Adolescent Health* 12: 434–42.

Slattery, M. (1991) 'Adolescents' knowledge and understanding of AIDS related concepts', paper given at the International Conference on Health Education, Helsinki, July.

Sloane, B., and Zimmer, C. (1993) 'The power of peer health education', *Journal of American College Health* 41: 241–5.

Slonim-Nevo, V. (1992) 'First pre-marital intercourse among Mexican Amer-

164   *Youth, AIDS, and STDs*

ican and Anglo-American adolescent women', *Journal of Adolescent Research* 7: 332–51.

Smith, A.M.A., Rosenthal, D.A., and Tesoriero, A. (1995) 'Adolescents and sexually transmissible diseases: patterns of knowledge in Victorian high schools', *Venereology* 8: 83–8.

Sobo, E.J. (1993) 'Inner city women and AIDS: the psycho-social benefits of unsafe sex', *Culture, Medicine and Psychiatry* 17: 455–85.

Sondheimer, D.L. (1992) 'HIV infection and disease among homeless adolescents', in R.J. DiClemente (ed.) *Adolescents and AIDS: A Generation in Jeopardy*, Newbury Park, Calif.: Sage.

Sonenstein, F., Pleck, J., and Ku, L. (1989) 'Sexual activity, condom use and AIDS awareness among adolescent males', *Family Planning Perspectives* 21: 152–8.

Spanier, G.B. (1976) 'Formal and informal sex education as determinants of premarital sexual behavior', *Archives of Sexual Behavior* 5: 39–67.

Spencer, L., Faulkner, A., and Keegan, J. (1988) *Talking About Sex: Asking the Public About Sexual Behaviour and Attitudes*, London: Social and Community Planning Research.

Spitzer, P.G., and Weiner, N.J. (1989) 'Transmission of HIV infection from a woman to a man by oral sex', *New England Journal of Medicine* 320: 251.

Springer, E. (1992) 'Reflections on women and HIV/AIDS in New York City and United States', in J. Bury, V. Morrison, and S. McLachlan (eds) *Working with Women and AIDS*, London: Routledge.

Stancombe, L. (1994) *Qualitative Research Findings on Young Heterosexuals: The 1994 Communication Environment in the Context of Sexually Transmitted Diseases Including HIV/AIDS*, Report to Research and Marketing Group Public Affairs Branch, Canberra, Australia.

Stevenson, E. (ed.) (1993) *Surveillance of Sexually Transmissible Diseases in Victoria 1992*, Victoria: AIDS/STD Unit, Department of Health and Community Services Victoria.

Stevenson, E., Gertig, D., Crofts, N., Sherrard, J., Forsyth, J., and Breschkin, A. (1992) 'Three potential spectres of youth: chlamydia, gonorrhoea and HIV in Victorian youth, January 1991 to June 1992', paper given at the Australian Scientific Congress on Sexually Transmissible Diseases, Sydney, November.

Stoller, E.J., and Rutherford, G.W. (1989) 'Evaluation of AIDS prevention and control programs', *AIDS* 3: 289–96.

Strunin, L., and Hingson, R. (1987) 'Acquired immune deficiency syndrome and adolescents: knowledge, beliefs, attitudes and behaviours', *Pediatrics* 79: 825–8.

Tacey, D. (1994) 'The psychology of adolescence, or, male development in a dysfunctional society', unpublished report, School of English, La Trobe University, Melbourne, Australia.

Tanfer, K., Grady, W.R., Klepinger, D.H., and Billy, J.O. (1991) 'Condom use among U.S. men', *Family Planning Perspectives* 25: 61–6.

Taylor, S.E., Lichtman, R.R., and Wood, J.V. (1984) 'Attributions, beliefs about control and adjustment to breast cancer', *Journal of Personality and Social Psychology* 46: 489–502.

Teichman, M., Barnea, Z., and Ravav, G. (1989) 'Personality and substance abuse among adolescents: a longitudinal study', *British Journal of Addiction* 84: 181–90.

Thomson, K. (1992) 'Being positive', in J. Bury, V. Morrison and S. McLachlan (eds) *Working with Women and AIDS*, London: Routledge.

Timko, C., and Janoff-Bulman, R. (1985) 'Attributions, vulnerability, and psychosocial adjustment: the case of breast cancer', *Health Psychology* 4: 521–44.

Tobler, N.S. (1986) 'Meta-analysis of 143 adolescent drug prevention programs: quantitative outcome results of program participants compared to control or comparison groups', *Journal of Drug Issues* 16: 537–67.

Traen, B., Lewin, B., and Sundet, J.N. (1992) 'Use of birth control pills and condoms among 17–19–year-old adolescents in Norway: contraceptive versus protective behaviour?', *AIDS Care* 4: 371–80.

Tross, S., and Hirsch, D. (1988) 'Psychological distress and neuropsychological complications of HIV and AIDS', *American Psychologist* 43: 929–34.

Turtle, A.M., Ford, B., Habgood, R., Grant, M., Bekiaris, J., Constantinou, C., Macek, M., and Polyzoidis, H. (1989) 'AIDS related beliefs and behaviours of Australian university students', *The Medical Journal of Australia* 150: 371–6.

Udry, J.R. (1985) 'Androgenic hormones motivate serum sexual behavior in boys', *Fertility and Sterility* 43: 90–4.

—— (1988) 'Biological predispositions and social control in adolescent sexual behavior', *American Sociological Review* 53: 709–22.

Udry, J.R., and Billy, J.O.G. (1987) 'Initiation of coitus in early adolescence', *American Sociological Review* 52: 841–55.

Uribe, V., and Harbeck, K. (1992) 'Addressing the needs of lesbian, gay and bisexual youth: the origins of PROJECT 10 and school-based intervention', in K.M. Harbeck (ed.) *Coming Out of the Classroom Closet: Gay and Lesbian Students, Teachers and Curricula*, New York: The Harvard Press.

Van de Perre, P., Jacobs, D., and Sprecher-Goldberger, S. (1987) 'The latex condom, an efficient barrier against sexual transmission of AIDS-related viruses', *AIDS* 1: 49–52.

Vanwesenbeeck, I., de Graaf, R., van Zessen, G., Straver, C.J., and Visser, J.H. (1993) 'Protection styles of prostitutes' clients: intentions, behavior, and considerations in relation to AIDS', *Journal of Sex Education and Therapy* 19: 79–92.

Victorian Government Department of Health and Community Services (1993) *Are You at Risk for STDs? A Simple Guide to Understanding and Preventing Sexually Transmissible Diseases*, Melbourne: Victorian Government Department of Health and Community Services.

Waldby, C., Kippax, S., and Crawford, J. (1990) 'Theory in the bedroom: a report from the Macquarie University AIDS and Heterosexuality Project', *Australian Journal of Social Issues* 25: 177–85.

Wasserheit, J.N. (1992) 'Interrelationships between human immunodeficiency virus infection and other sexually transmitted diseases', *Sexually Transmitted Diseases* 19: 61–77.

Wasserheit, J.N., Aral, S.O., and Holmes, K.K. (eds) (1991) *Research Issues in Human Behaviour and Sexually Transmitted Diseases in the AIDS Era*, Washington, DC: American Society for Microbiology.

Waters, L. (1992) 'The nature and development of preadolescents' and adolescents' understanding of HIV/AIDS', unpublished thesis, Department of Psychology, University of Melbourne, Melbourne, Australia.

Waugh, M.A. (1990) 'History of clinical developments in sexually transmitted diseases', in K.K. Holmes, P-A. Mardh, P.F. Sparling, P.J. Wiesner, W. Cates, S.M. Lemon, and W.E. Stamm (eds) *Sexually Transmitted Disease*, 2nd edn, New York: McGraw Hill.

Weber, F.T., Elfenbein, D.S., Richards, N.L., Davis, A.B., and Thomas, J.T. (1989) 'Early sexual activity of delinquent adolescents', *Journal of Adolescent Health Care* 10: 398–403.

Weeks, J. (1985) *Sexuality and its Discontents*, London: Routledge & Kegan Paul.

Weinstein, N.D. (1984) 'Why it won't happen to me: perceptions of risk factors and susceptibility', *Health Psychology* 3: 431–57.

Weisberg, E., North, P., and Buxton, M. (1992) 'Sexual activity and condom use in high school students', *The Medical Journal of Australia* 156: 612–3.

Weisenberg, M., Kegeles, S.S., and Lund, A.K. (1980) 'Children's health beliefs and acceptance of a dental preventive activity', *Journal of Health and Social Behavior* 21: 59–74.

Weissman, C., Nathanson, C., Ensminger, M., Robinson, J., and Plitcha, S. (1989) 'AIDS knowledge, perceived risk, and prevention among adolescent clients attending a family planning clinic', *Family Planning Perspectives* 21: 213–7.

Weitz, R. (1989) 'Uncertainty and the lives of persons with AIDS', *Journal of Health and Social Behavior* 30: 270–81.

Wellings, L. (1994) 'It ain't a level playing field...', *National AIDS Bulletin* 8(7): 8–9.

Wells, J. (1992) 'Public policy perspectives on HIV Education', in R.J. DiClemente (ed.) *Adolescents and AIDS: A Generation in Jeopardy*, Newbury Park, Calif.: Sage.

Whitehead, B.D. (1994) 'The failure of sex education', *The Atlantic Monthly*, October: 55–78.

WHO (1981) *Global Strategy for Health for All by the Year 2000*, Geneva: World Health Organization.

—— (1986) *Ottawa Charter for Health Promotion*, Geneva: World Health Organization.

—— (1990) 'AIDS and the status of women – challenges and perspectives for the 1990s', in *WHO Features No.149*, Geneva: World Health Organization.

Wicklund, B.M., and Jackson, M.A. (1992) 'Coping with AIDS in hemophilia', in P.I. Ahmed (ed.) *Living and Dying with AIDS*, New York: Plenum Press.

Wight, D. (1992) 'Impediments to safer heterosexual sex: a review of research with young people', *AIDS Care* 4: 11–21.

Wildavsky, A. (1988) *Searching for Safety*, New Brunswick: Transaction Books.

Wilders, S., and MacCallum, M. (1990) *Research Report: Women and AIDS*, Report to the Department of Community Services and Health, Canberra, Australia.

Wille, A. (1995) 'Affirming diversity', *HEAV Quarterly*, Summer 95: 14–9.

Williams, T. (1957) *A Streetcar Named Desire*, London: Secker & Warburg.

Wodak, A. (1995) 'Needle exchange and bleach distribution programmes: the Australian experience', *The International Journal of Drug Policy* 6: 46–57.

Worth, D. (1989) 'Sexual decision making and AIDS: why condom promotion

among vulnerable women is likely to fail', *Studies in Family Planning* 20: 297–307.
Wright, B. (1990) 'Student perceptions of AIDS: seriousness and personal risk assessments', unpublished manuscript, University of Queensland.
Wright, S.M., Gabb, R.G., and Ryan, M.M. (1991) 'Reproductive health: knowledge, attitudes and needs of adolescents', *The Medical Journal of Australia* 155: 325–8.
Wyn, J. (1993) *Young Women's Health: The Challenge of Sexually Transmitted Diseases*, Working Paper no. 8, Melbourne, Youth Research Centre.
Wyn, J., and Stewart, F. (1991) *Young Women and Sexually Transmitted Diseases*, Working Paper no. 7, Melbourne, Youth Research Centre.
Yesmont, G.A. (1992) 'The relationship of assertiveness to college students' safer sex behaviors', *Adolescence* 27: 253–72.
Youth Policy Development Council (1987) *Health for Youth Final Report: Policies and Strategies*, Melbourne: Youth Policy Development Council.
Zelnick, M., Kantner, J., and Ford, K. (1981) *Sex and Pregnancy in Adolescence*, Beverly Hills, Calif.: Sage.
Zimet, G.D., Hillier, S.A., Anglin, T.M., Ellick, E.M., Krowchuk, D.P., and Williams P. (1991) 'Knowing someone with AIDS: the impact on adolescents', *Journal of Pediatric Psychology* 16: 287–94.
Zuckerman, M. (1979) *Sensation Seeking: Beyond the Optimal Level of Arousal*, Hillsdale, NJ: Lawrence Erlbaum Associates.
—— (1983) 'A biological theory of sensation seeking', in M. Zuckerman (ed.) *Biological Bases of Sensation Seeking, Impulsivity, and Anxiety*, Hillsdale, NJ: Lawrence Erlbaum Associates.

Index

Abbott, S. 29, 49, 74
Abraham, C. 42, 43, 114, 115
Abrams, D. 44, 49
acquired immune deficiency
   syndrome *see* AIDS
Adelman, M.B. 86, 87
Adimara, A.A. 3, 9, 14
Adler, N. 56
Africa 13
age of consent 101
AIDS 8; bereavement 136;
   psychiatric disorders 136–7; Risk
   Reduction Model 59–60; women
   138–40; *see also* HIV/AIDS
AIDS-related complex (ARC) 8
Ajzen, I. 41, 57, 58, 59, 111
Altman, D. 76, 95
anal sex 20–1; age of consent 101;
   non-use of condoms 29
Anderson, M.D. 123
Andre, T. 35, 42
Andrucci, G.L. 62
Aneshensel, C.S. 18
anger 130
Anns, M. 128, 129, 130, 131, 132
anxiety 130
Aral, S.O. 11, 14
Asia 13
assertiveness 61–2, 79–80
Australia: condom use 28–9;
   epidemiology 12–13; ethnic
   groups 22–3; homeless young
   people 31; knowledge of HIV/
   AIDS 35–6; knowledge of STDs
   39; national HIV/AIDS policy

94–9, 145; number of partners 24;
   sexual debut 18

Baldo, M. 124
Bamford, E.J. 105–6
Bandura, A. 61
Barker, L.F. 137
Barling, N. 50
Barnard, M. 30
Bartlett, J.G. 140
Bauman, K. 18
Becker, M.H. 56, 61
Bell, D. 35, 42
Benton, J.M. 39
bereavement 136
Billy, J.O.G. 66
bisexuality 21–2
Blaney, N.T. 137
Blewett, Neal 95
Boldero, J.M. 36, 50, 58, 82
Bormann, L. 35, 42
Bowler, S. 35, 48
Boyer, C.B. 35
Brady, M. 32
Breakwell, G.M. 17, 21, 28, 29, 60
breast feeding 10, 140
Britain: condom use 28; intravenous
   drug users 30; sexual debut 17
Brookman, R.R. 14
Brooks-Gunn, J. 18
Brown, N. 64
Buhrich, N. 136
Bury, J.K. 13, 138, 139, 140
Buzwell, S. 19, 24, 25, 49, 65

Carmichael, I. 92

Cass, V.C. 133
casual sex 16; condom use 29
Catania, J.A. 59
Cates, W. 13
cervical cancer 9–10
Chaikin, A. 33
Chapman, S. 48
Chassin, L. 63
Chilman, C.S. 51
Chlamydia trachomatis infections 4–5;
  epidemiology 12; knowledge
  about 39–40; neonatal eye
  infections 10
Christenson, G.M. 123
Cline, R. 32, 82, 84
Cochran, S.D. 33
Coleman, J.C. 19
Coles, P. 137
Coles, R. 20
Collis, F. 41, 109
communication 81–3
condoms: attitudes to 48–51, 52;
  campaigns 49; and contraception
  51, 78, 83–4; intended use 49–50,
  57–9; intravenous drug users 30;
  and knowledge about HIV/AIDS
  36; negative implications of
  carrying 48–9, 78; non-use 26–9,
  82–3, 85; peer education 112; in
  prisons 31–2; and prostitution 31;
  psychosocial factors 72–3;
  reliability 88; talking about 81–3
confidentiality 99–100
Connell, R.W. 111
conspiracy theories 86
contact tracing 14, 100
Contagious Diseases Bill (1864) 2
contraception 51, 78, 83–4
Corey, L. 5
Crawford, J. 29, 35, 36, 44, 49

Dank, B.M. 22
Darling, C.A. 69, 108
David, H.P. 124
Davidson, A.R. 56
Dean, L. 136
De Graaf, R. 88
depression 130
Derelega, V.J. 33
Des Jarlais, D.C. 102

Devaney, B.L. 18
Dew, M.A. 136
DiClemente, R.J. 13, 26, 35, 37, 50
discrimination 101–4, 132
dishonesty 33
Donald, M. 51
Dryfoos, J. 54, 124
Dunne, M. 18, 28, 35, 40, 41, 43, 111,
  112, 123
Dusek, J.B. 18, 19

education 105–25, 146–8; aims 120–2;
  history 105–7; homosexual men
  121–2; mass media 41–2, 115–18;
  opportunistic 114–15; by parents
  41, 107–10; peer education 43–4,
  110–14; programmes 41–4, 72;
  school-based 118–25
Ehrhardt, A.A. 121, 122, 124, 125
Elkind, D. 65
Ellickson, P.L. 12
Elliott, G. 53
epidemiology 11–14
Erikson, E. 126
ethnic groups 22–3

Fahey, J. 117
faithfulness 25–6
fantasies 87
Farmer, P. 86
fatalism 50, 86
Faulstich, M.E. 129
Feacham, R.G.A. 145
Feldman, S.S. 53, 64
Fennell, R. 111
Ferrara, A.J. 128
Fife-Schaw, C. 17, 21, 28, 29, 60
Fine, M. 87
Finkbeiner, A.K. 140
First World War 2
Fishbein, M. 41, 57, 59, 111
Forrest, D.J. 118
Foucault, M. 106
Frankham, J. 83
Fullilove, R.E. 143
Furstenberg, F.F. 18

Galligan, R. 74, 78, 89
Gallois, C. 29, 36, 44, 49
Garland, S.M. 12

gay-related immune deficiency
  (GRID) 7; *see also* AIDS; HIV/
  AIDS
gender-role expectations 76–80;
  mass media 116–17
genital herpes 5–6; emotional
  aspects 142; epidemiology 12–13;
  knowledge about 39–40; mother-
  to-child infection 10
genital warts 6; cervical cancer 9–10;
  differential diagnosis 15;
  epidemiology 12–13; knowledge
  about 40; mother-to-child
  infection 10
Gerety, R.J. 137
Geringer, W.M. 49
Getty, A. 111
Gilbert, P. 116
Glaun, D. 38
Glunt, E.K. 103
Goggin, M. 22, 77, 126
Gold, R. 80, 81, 82, 83, 85
Goldman, J.D.G. 17, 18, 19
Goldman, R.J. 17, 18, 19
gonorrhoea 4; epidemiology 12;
  history 2–3; and HIV infection 9;
  knowledge about 40; neonatal eye
  infections 10
Grant, D. 128, 129, 130, 131, 132
Greig, R. 36
Griffin, H. 83
Grimes, D.A. 53
Gullone, E. 68
Gunn, D. 71
Gurien, R. 83–4
Guyomard, P. 71

Hadley, S. 61–2
haemophiliacs 127, 137–8
Haffner, D. 14
Hale, R.W. 145
Hall, L. 101
Harbeck, K. 122, 125
Harris, M.B. 42, 115
Hart, G. 12
Hayes, C.D. 18
Health Belief Model 56–7
health education *see* education
health professionals 43–4
Hendry, L. 19

Henry, S. 19
hepatitis B 6–7; epidemiology 12;
  mother-to-child infection 10
Herek, G.M. 102, 103
herpes simplex virus *see* genital
  herpes
Hersch, P. 31
Hicks, M.W. 69, 108
Hingson, R. 27, 35, 36, 56
Hirsch, D. 136
HIV/AIDS: Australian national
  policy 94–9, 145; condom use
  27–8; coping 131–8;
  discrimination 101–4, 132;
  epidemiology 13–14; and
  gonorrhoea 9; haemophiliacs 127,
  137–8; homosexual men 127,
  133–6; intravenous drug users
  127; knowledge about 35–9, 60–2;
  living with the disease 126–43;
  mother-to-child infection 10,
  139–40; and other STDs 3, 9;
  response to diagnosis 128–31; risk
  perception 44–7; sources of
  information 40–4; stereotypes
  45–6, 84–5; symptoms 7–9; testing
  8, 129; transmission through
  blood 36, 37; transmission by oral
  sex 20; treatment 8;
  understanding 37–9; *see also* AIDS
Hodgson, J. 48
Hofferth, S.L. 17, 18
Holland, J. 49, 73, 78, 83, 136
Holmes, K.K. 3, 7, 11, 14
homeless young people: anal sex 21;
  intravenous drug use 31;
  knowledge of HIV/AIDS 36;
  prostitution 31; risk behaviour 37;
  risk perception 44; sexual activity
  24; unsafe sex 30–2
homosexual men: condom non-use
  82–3, 85; discrimination 101;
  education 121–2; hepatitis B 7;
  HIV-positive 127, 133–6;
  negotiated safety 76; peer
  education 111
homosexuality: exclusivity 22;
  experimentation with 21–2
Howard, J. 28
Hubley, K.S. 18

human immunodeficiency virus *see* HIV/AIDS
human papilloma virus *see* genital warts
Hunter, B. 101

identity formation 126–7
infertility 9
Ingham, R. 82, 83
Internet 118, 134
intravenous drug users: condom use 30; harm minimisation 96–8; HIV-positive 127; homeless young people 31; peer education 111; sexual debut 19
invulnerability 44–5, 65, 84–5
Irwin, C.E. 54, 66, 67, 68, 111

Jaccard, J. 56
Jackson, A. 111
Jackson, M.A. 137
Janoff-Bulman, R. 143
Jessor, R. 46, 54, 66
Jessor, S.L. 46, 54, 66
Johnson, A.M. 17, 20, 21, 22, 23, 28
Johnson, V. 81
Jones, R.B. 4, 5, 7, 10
Joseph, J.G. 56, 61

Kashima, Y. 48, 50
Katz, S. 95
Kegeles, S. 35, 36, 49, 145
Keller, S.E. 36
Kent, V. 78, 81, 83
King, A. 31
Kinsey, A.C. 17
Kippax, S. 78, 79, 111, 117
Kirby, D. 115, 119, 123, 124, 125
Klee, H. 30
Klitsch, M. 49
Koopman, C. 37
Kovacs, G.T. 12
Ku, L. 145
Kubler-Ross, E. 133, 135

Leap, N. 101
Lee, C. 81
Lemon, S.M. 7
Lenehan, Lynton, Bloom & Blaxland 48

Levenson, M.R. 62
Levitt, M.Z. 60, 62, 63, 67, 69
Lhuede, D. 21, 24, 29, 31, 44
lies 33
liver disease 6–7
Louie, R. 19, 30
love 73–6
Loxley, W. 30
Lucke, J. 45

MacCallum, M. 42, 114, 123
McCamish, M. 36, 44
McKeganey, N. 30
McKenzie, J. 98
McLeod, J. 97
McRobbie, A. 116
Madden, T.J. 41, 58, 59, 111
Mannison, M. 121
mass media 41–2, 115–18
Masters, W. 81
Matthews, B.R. 36, 44
Mays, V.M. 33
media 41–2, 115–18
mental health 11, 140–1; AIDS patients 136–7
Mertz, G.J. 6
Metzler, C.W. 54
Millstein, S.G. 66, 67, 111
Mindel, A. 4, 5, 6
Minichiello, V. 39, 40
Misson, R. 116, 118
Mitchell, A. 117, 119
monogamy 25–6, 73–6
Moore, S.M. 19, 21, 23–5, 29, 31, 40–1, 44–7, 49–50, 54, 63, 65, 68–9, 73, 76, 81, 84, 86–7, 108–9, 111, 114, 129, 142, 144
Morris, R.E. 31, 32
Morrison, D. 48, 51
mortality 53

Neisseria gonorrhoea see gonorrhoea
Neustatter, W.L. 101
Newbold, J.E. 7
Newcomer, S.J. 18, 20
Noack, P. 63
non-specific urethritis 12
Nott, P. 97

O'Campo, P. 143

O'Connell, J.K. 56
O'Donnell, M. 111
O'Keefe, T. 135, 136, 141
Ollis, D. 90, 120
Omelczuk, S. 100
oral sex 20
Oriel, D. 6
Orr, D.P. 36
Ottawa Charter for Health
    Promotion 91, 110
Ovenden, P. 30

Palmer, G. 95
parents: as information-givers 41,
    107–10; sexual behaviour 64,
    108–9; values 108, 110
Parkes, Dr 2
partners: changing 23–4; condoms
    and lack of trust 48–9, 78; contact
    tracing 14, 100; HIV-positive 132;
    judgements 27, 80–1; past history
    discussion 32–3, 82
Patton, W. 121
Peart, R. 121
peer education 43–4, 110–14
pelvic inflammatory disease 9;
    epidemiology 12
personality 62–3
Pleck, J.H. 79
Plummer, D. 3, 8, 9, 10, 15
Porter, R. 101
Potter, J. 117
pregnancy 10, 139–40
premarital sex 16–19; parents'
    influence 108–9; and religion 18,
    92, 106
prevention: health education *see*
    education; policies 90–104
prisons 31–2; risk behaviour 37
prostitutes 2–3; homeless young
    people 31
psychiatric disorders *see* mental
    health
Psychosocial Foundations Model
    60–6
public health 90–104
Pyett, P. 142

radio, talk-back shows 117, 118
Raphael, B. 36

recklessness 65–6
Reiser, C. 142
relationship dysfunction 10–11
religious beliefs 18, 92, 106
Reulbach, W. 128
Richard, R. 36, 50
Richie, N. 111
Rickert, V.I. 112
risk 53–71; AIDS Risk Reduction
    Model 59–60; homeless young
    people 37, 44; management
    strategies 61–2; partner selection
    32–3; perceptions of 44–7, 67–9;
    recklessness 65–6; youth as risk
    factor 12–14
rites of passage 67
Roberts, C. 20
Robinson, J. 51
Robinson, R. 97
Rogel, J. 18
Rosenstock, I.M. 56
Rosenthal, D.A. 18–25, 28–9, 35–47,
    49–50, 54, 56, 58, 62–3, 65, 69, 73–6,
    81, 84, 86–7, 108–9, 111–12, 114–15,
    119, 129, 142, 144–5
Ross, M.W. 97, 130, 131, 133, 134
Rotheram-Borus, M.J. 35, 37
Rutherford, G.W. 111

safe sex 14, 145–6; campaigns 49;
    condoms *see* condoms; HIV-
    infected individuals 132; and
    knowledge about HIV/AIDS
    36–7; *see also* unsafe sex
St Lawrence, J.S. 49
Schmidt, G. 124
Schoenbaum, E.E. 139
Schofield, M. 78
schools 118–25
Scott, A. 83
Sears, J.T. 121
Second World War 2–3
self-efficacy 61–2
sensation seeking trait 62
serial monogamy 26
service accessibility 99–100
sex drive 76–80
sex education *see* education
sex hormones 66
sexual abuse 19

Sexual Attitudes and Lifestyles survey 17
sexual behaviour 16–34; ethnic groups 22–3; and knowledge 51–2; likes and dislikes 23; number of partners 23–4; parents' influence 64, 108–9; prepubertal sex 19; risk taking *see* risk; variety of practices 20–3
sexual debut 17–19
sexual dysfunction 10–11
sexual orientation 21–2; *see also* homosexual men; homosexuality
sexually transmitted diseases (STDs): attitudes to 47–8; bacterial 3; complications 9–11; diagnosis 15; epidemiology 11–14; history 1–3; and HIV/AIDS 3, 9; knowledge of 39–40; living with 141–3; risk perception 44–7; sources of information 40–4; symptoms 3–9; treatment 14–15; vaccines 3; viral 3
Shepherd, H. 145
Short, R.V. 9, 12, 44
Short, S. 95
Silbereisen, R.K. 63
Silverman, J. 118
situational judgements 27
Slap, B. 111
Slattery, M. 37, 42
Sloane, B. 111
Slonim-Nevo, V. 18
Smith, A.M.A. 2, 39, 42–3, 46, 108, 112, 114–15, 119, 123
Sobo, E.J. 72–3, 74, 77, 83, 86
sociocultural variables 63–5
soldiers 2
Sondheimer, D.L. 30, 31
Sonenstein, F. 35
Spanier, G.B. 18
Spencer, L. 81
Spitzer, P.G. 20
Springer, E. 138
Stancombe, L. 20, 41, 42, 48, 115
stereotypes 45–6, 72–89
Stevenson, E. 12
Stewart, F. 36, 39, 125
Stokes, G. 20
Stoller, E.J. 111

Stronach, I. 83
Strunin, L. 27, 35
support groups 134
Sweden 17
syphilis: history 1–3; knowledge about 39–40; mother-to-child infection 10

Tacey, D. 67
Tanfer, K. 51
Taylor, S. 116
Taylor, S.E. 143
Teichman, M. 62
Terry, D. 74, 78, 89
Theory of Reasoned Action 57–9
Thomson, K. 139
Timko, C. 143
Traen, B. 51
Tross, S. 136
True Love Waits campaign 18–19
trust 73–6, 84; and condom use 48–9, 78
Turtle, A.M. 21, 29, 35, 36, 37

Udry, J.R. 18, 20, 66
United States: condom use 27–8; epidemiology 12–13; knowledge of HIV/AIDS 35–6; prevention policy 93; prisoners 32; sexual debut 17–18
unsafe sex 26–32, 51–2; psychosocial factors 72–89; *see also* safe sex
Uribe, V. 122, 125

Van de Perre, P. 88
Van der Pligt, J. 36, 50
Vanwesenbeeck, I. 88
venereal disease 1–3
venturesomeness 63
verbal communication 81–3

Waldby, C. 78
Walker, I. 135, 136, 141
warts *see* genital warts
Wasserheit, J.N. 3, 4–5, 7, 9–10, 14, 125
Waugh, M.A. 1
Weber, F.T. 19
Weeks, J. 101
Weiner, N.J. 20

Weinstein, N.D. 45, 66
Weisberg, E. 28
Weisenberg, M. 56
Weissman, C. 36
Weitz, R. 129
Wellings, L. 102
Wells, J. 92
Wetherall, M. 117
Whitehead, B.D. 122
Wicklund, B.M. 137
Wight, D. 73, 78, 81, 82
Wildavsky, A. 86
Wilders, S. 42, 114, 123
Wille, A. 122
Williams, T. 81
withdrawal 21

Wodak, A. 94, 97
women with AIDS 138–40
World Health Organization 91, 104
Worth, D. 49
Wright, B. 44
Wright, S.M. 39, 41, 43
Wyn, J. 29, 36, 39, 42, 125

Yesmont, G.A. 61, 62

Zelnick, M. 18
Zidovudine 8
Zimet, G.D. 84
Zimmer, C. 111
Zuckerman, M. 62